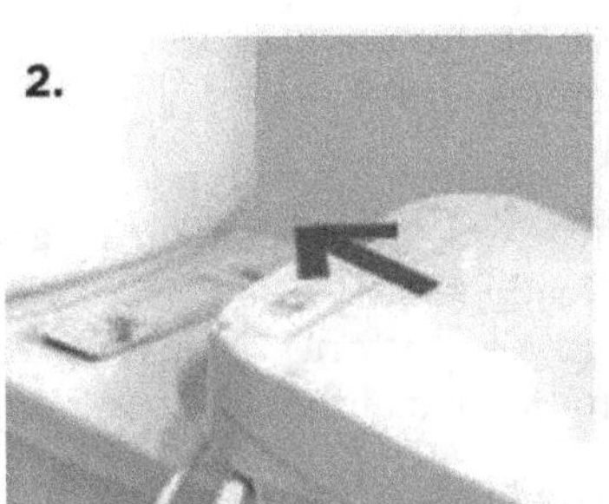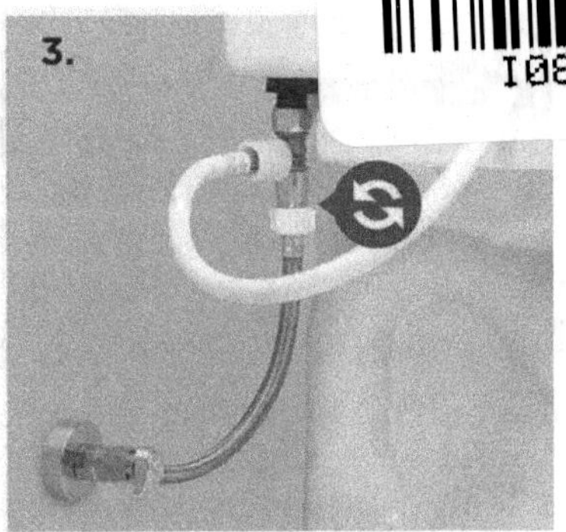

The Bidet

Everything There is to Know
From the First and only Book on the Bidet
An Elegant Solution for Comfort, Health,
Happiness, Ecology, and Economy
The Topic No One Talks About,
The Device That Can Save Your Life

Second Edition

William L. Bruneau

Photo Credits and any descriptions are at the back of this book just after **References.** Front cover: Darling milieu ca. 2005

This is a solo work: thought, researched, written, edited, typeset all by myself. Inevitably in such a solo work some mistakes have been made and I would appreciate any corrections from my readers. My wife Betsy's excellent discernment and advice were essential to this effort. Kudos to Amazon for making printing on demand a reality, giving novice authors a "free" opportunity.

My original intention in writing this book was as a literary work and a cultural story that would be a slightly risqué but an enjoyable read. It contains many colorful but telling anecdotes about how bidets are perceived and used around the world; none of them are verifiable, most have been culled from internet chat groups, and hopefully capture our societal feelings about bidets, and the world viewpoint. Then the facts got in the way; we have painted ourselves into a corner culturally and must have the courage to change, and largely walk away from TP.

Disclaimer

This book is intended to give you a broad consumer understanding and knowledge of bidets. This book surveys what bidets are: their forms, generally how they work, what possible benefits they may offer, and how they are used. This book also offers a major critique of our dominant industrial method of disposing of our bodily wastes (flush toilets and toilet paper), using scant publicly available government and commercial sources from the internet for often dubious verification. Industry information, especially about pollution, is unobtainable (or unaffordable) so I have had to go to secondary or tertiary sources for data. I have felt compelled to use sources that are less than perfect. The use of this information and the conclusions I have drawn may have to change with better information, so take this information with "a grain of salt".

This book periodically draws on statistics and information that may be quite questionable, and text and information contained in this book may come to conclusions that may be wrong. While this book cites a number of scientific studies, my interpretation may be tenuous, faulty or overly enthusiastic. Most of the information in this book, and most particularly the Health chapter, should be considered offering preliminary and perhaps suspect information. Users are therefore reminded to seek the advice of their health provider in relation to anything mentioned in this book; **under no circumstances does this book offer medical advice.** Hopefully it raises some issues to bring up with your health care providers, though it is always your health care provider who should judge its correctness for your health. Topics such as bidet assembly may be overly simplistic, and are not a replacement for the manufacturer's complete directions. **Disclaimer continues on page 198.**

Disclaimer continues on page 198.

Copyright 2004-2020, William Bruneau
WB/P: William Bruneau, Publisher
Contact: bbruneauca@gmail.com
Original Library of Congress number LCCN: 2004096271
Original   ISBN: 0-9748799-0-8
Second Edition ISBN: 9781693610936

Table Of Contents

Ecology of the Bidet

Cleaning With A Bidet

Water and the Bidet

Toilet Paper vs. Environment

Economic Costs of TP Production

Manufacturers don't use all types of trees to make paper. Toilet paper is generally made from "virgin" paper, using a combination of softwood and hardwood trees (a combination of approx, 70% hardwood and 30% softwood). Other materials for final product of toilet paper include water, chemicals and bleaches.[53]

Toilet Paper Environment

Toilet Paper Un-Health

Toilet Paper Ecology

Toilet Paper Sociology

Appendices

Introduction

Fifteen years ago my first edition of **The Bidet** was the first book on that topic, ever. It was the first book, and probably the first publication on the bidet ever in our Library of Congress. It became known in the bidet biz as "the bidet bible" for the completeness of its information and the available peer-review research. It also featured personal, scatological, and humorous anecdotes about the bidet, and how we relate to it. Please note that some of the quotes are quite raw.

This second edition has evolved into two compelling books: the first book is still about bidets, their health benefits, medical benefits, and their sheer enjoyment and cleanliness. I have even managed to expand on the bidet humor.

This latest edition that highlights the joys and benefits of the bidet was as fun to put together as the first edition. The humor and the play is still there around the unmentionable acts that each of us perform every day. Medicine and science have validated even more benefits of the bidet, while more anecdotes reveal the very personal relationships people have with their bidet.

The ensuing 15 years has seen the technological side of the bidet benefit from the growth of the computer and microprocessors. What I call "toilet seat bidets" (TSB) have essentially become the dedicated personal robots of the bathroom. They not only make your defecation as pleasant as possible; they can now potentially provide a myriad of health checks at the same time.

[French bidet] I bathed my baby in one in Italy. There was no tub in the hotel, and she just fit. During a year in Paris, we used ours for washing smalls and feet, as well as the intended parts. Our flat had only one toilet for four people, and I will admit that my husband and son used it as a urinal occasionally. I miss it terribly.[23]

The second half of this book is a critique and condemnation of our current method of processing our bodily wastes, particularly with TP. My argument is that bidets are a huge and critical part of a sustainable solution to our TP crisis; and we now have a very serious environmental crisis over soft fluffy TP.

The bidet part of this book was fun to write, the facts and details of our evolving and ensuing TP disaster were not. We are facing multiple ecologic disasters caused by our wanton and relentless use of TP, wipes, disposable diapers (young and old), and so on. It is a good story and we are ripe for a change.

The rise of our TP use and municipal septic systems is a fascinating story of a system that worked well for us three hundred years ago, with a population that was much much smaller and less dense than today. This system does not work well with mega-million population densities, nor with 7 billion people all wanting "a better life". We have finite amounts of water, arable land, harvestable trees, and landfill space in the world, and there are not enough resources for everyone to have their TP. If most of us convert to bidets the problem becomes irrelevant.

I tried to present quotes in **this special font** but not always. Sometimes a quote simply did not fit otherwise. Where I had extra space I often randomly dropped in quotes or pictures. Photo Credits and descriptions are just after **References**.

An audio interview with my grand-daughter Clara a week after installing "a top end" bidet that had a warm seat and air dry along with multiple spray patterns and angles:

E: Grandpa Bill wants a response from you kids about what you think about our new bidet

C and A: (Double thumbs up)

E: Can you say it though? (everyone laughs)

C: (pause) I really like it.

E: You really like it. Why do you like it? What are the top three reasons why you really like the bidet?

C: (Whispers conspiratorially) It sprays you. You do not have to use toilet paper.

Emile and Stephanie (in chorus): Yeah.

E: And why is it so great to not have to have to use TP?

C: (Again whispers conspiratorially) No trees cut down. Yesss

S No trees cut down. Yeah.

E: Yeah

E: For how long do we have to not have to buy TP?

C: Forever.

E&S: Laugthter

C: But we do need...well for the bathroom downstairs.

S: Yes, the bathroom downstairs

A: (rolls something for awhile then stops)

Clara: Yeah. The bathroom downstairs...(pause)... but we will still need to cut down trees, but its a **lot less** trees (ending in a very hopeful tone).

E: Are there any other things you like about the bidet?

C: I like how it goes for a really long time and you can choose if you want to stop it now or like not stop it...(pause)..... and i like how it moves. you can press the move button and it like moves, and it kind of feels like a butt massage.

E and S: (laugh)

Stephanie (still laughing): "I like that too"

E: Is it fun to use?

C: Yes

Stephanie: "I think Atty's favorite thing is holding the remote

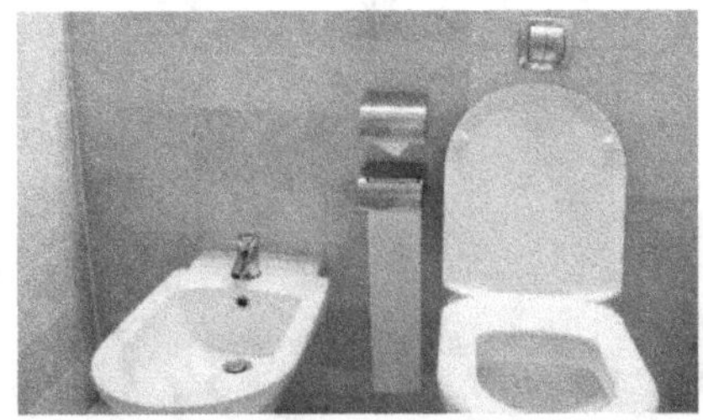 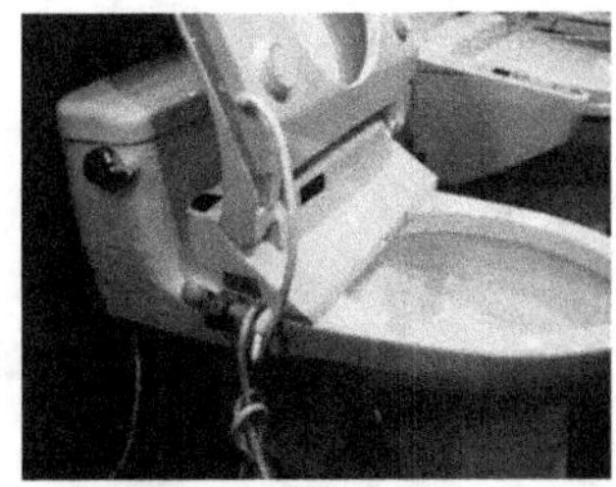

All About the Bidet

Some form of bidet is a familiar household device in much of the world, yet bidets are controversial in the English speaking West. A good way to begin this tale is with a description of the many forms of bidet but first a few quotes of bidet users.

I'm from Argentina, Bidets are installed on 100% of the houses around here, and even though not everyone uses it, it's far more hygienic than just using toilet paper. FAR MORE!....   I'm from Argentina too, where everybody has a bidet at home. I spent two years in Germany without using one and it was a terrible experience... only with TP i feel my ass was dirty all the time.... Hallo everybody ! Your conversation about bidet is very interesting to me! I am from Italy and I have to say I find it highly higenic. After living in England for some years, I realised that the rate of female genitalia diseases due to less higenic conditions (like cystitis) much higher that in Italy.[12]

I am not from the USA or a Latin country, where the people seems to believe toilet paper is unhygienic. In all my 53 years I have done well with toilet paper thank you. Bidets are rare in South Africa too. However, over the last 2 years I developed a condition where my bowels are not working properly and I need frequent trips to the loo and sometimes need washing not only in the butt crack but even into the rectum to bring relief. I just returned from a hotel with a bidet and found it very handy with the aim to install one at home.[216]

Krikeys! Is that what the low boy is for? First, I thought it might be a dedicated baby bath. So I washed my infant son in it for awhile but he outgrew it after a year or two. Then I thought it was a training toilet, the seat area was too large and so LDP kept falling in. Besides, at that point, he was so used to taking a bath in it that the wanted to get naked and jump in.[12]

To the idiot who thinks having a shower is cleaner: So you like washing your poop onto the floor you stand on? Lovely, I hope I don't have to share a bathroom with you. The bidet is designed for this, the shower isn't."....   I am in the trucking business. All of you have seen the picture of the 400 pound trucker with the Tee shirt that says "I Beat Bulimia". Well this fella needs to grow some longer arms so he can reach around his butt cheeks and clean himself after each dump. Nothing like the smell of a 400 pound ass to convince you of the merits of a bidet.[12]

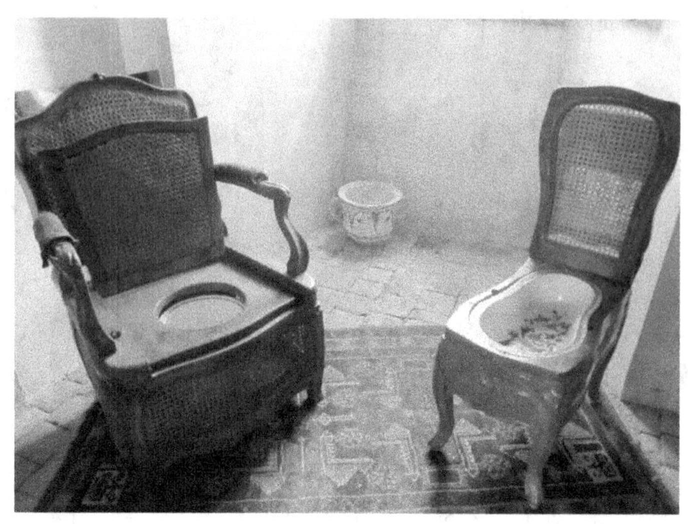

Different Kinds of Bidets

The last 60 years have seen the most revolutionary change ever in how we process our bodily wastes with the development of several devices to clean our derrieres more effectively; they are all generically called the bidet. Their commonality is that they use water to wash your derriere clean and need little or no toilet paper.

The functionality, usability and affordability of "the bidet" have soared. Many models can simply replace the toilet seat and attach to the toilet's water supply. These units are amazingly compact and modern materials make them very durable. With modern electronics you can have sophisticated digital controls.

This chapter discusses the different forms of the bidet. There is a lot to recommend any of these various forms of the bidet; and the monetary barrier to owning some form of this healthful device is minimal. Buying a cheap starter unit may satisfy your needs forever, or can allow you to realize what additional bidet functions suit your personal or family needs. The typical setup of each type of bidet is covered in **Setting Up The Bidet Unit** on page 92.

It is important at the outset to understand that there are many different types of bidets available for your use. Bidets use the same home water system and sewer lines that the flush toilet uses. They all use very little water to cleanse your perianal region, with limited or no need for toilet paper. They fall into certain categories defined by their physical shape and characteristics. You can choose a bidet that exactly fits your needs, and certainly your checkbook (remember you will save on TP). The categories below constantly are blurring; the new generation toilet seat bidets (I call them TSBs for short) used to be the only place to go for all the benefits of modern electronics, but that is no longer the situation. There is now little difference between classic/French bidets, and either can now be installed with much the same electronics. Portables can have electronics.

The (French) bidet is a low-set basin for cleansing with a cloth or sponge or rinsing with a built-in-spray. The basin or bowl is equipped with hot and cold water supplies and a pop-up valve to retain water in the bowl or to drain it when desired. The bidet is also provided with an integral douche or jet, operated when desired and directing a stream of column of water upward from the bottom of the bowl. This optional jet stream for certain purposes is an easier and cleaner method of ablution, to say nothing of its refreshing action. The entire apparatus is designed to maintain for the user a constant state of cleanliness of the various private parts. It is always installed beside the water closet or commode for easy accessibility.[182] [George Peck, MD, "In Praise of the Bidet" 1959]

Can someone recommend a (TSB) bidet?   I've had mine for five years now. Same brand. It is cheaply made of plastic, but I've had no issues with it. I put another one of my second bathroom. No issues either. Would buy again.... We got it in July of this year, paid ~$60 for it. It is a very simple one. I liked it because it looks almost exactly like a regular toilet seat. It's fine if you don't mind the lack of temperature control; which I was worried would be a big deal, and turns out so far it has not been an issue, we'll see after this winter if that holds true. No complaints about this unit; it does exactly what it is supposed to do. It's likely that we will spring for a more expensive & fancier one some day, maybe one with a warm-air dryer; but this one gets the job done....   My mom's basic Toto model is going on 20 years. My grandma had one that was much older than that....   The last time I went to Korea was in 2006 and almost every home bathroom had a bidet with a little remote at the side to choose different functions like spray my butthole, clean the bowl, blow my butt with warm air. That shit was glourious....   What about the handheld sprayer kinds? Those are honestly my fav from traveling around, and I would think any one you get would be BIFL. It's just a steel hose and sprayer, like you find on most kitchen sinks nowadays.[246]

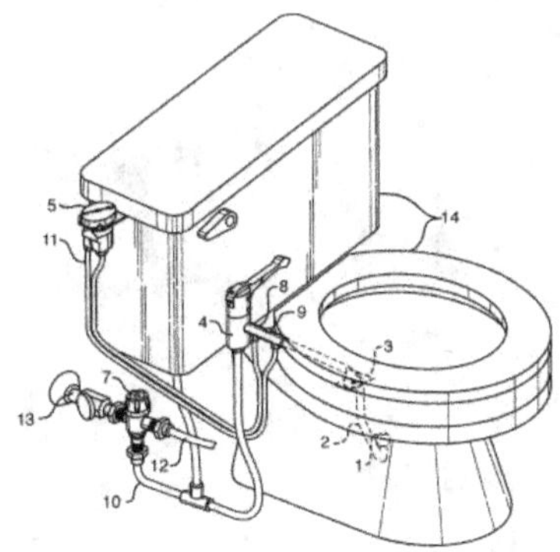

Bidet Identification

First of all a quick visual guide to the various forms of bidet, followed by a
detailed study of each type of bidet.

Floor Models

These are units the general size and shape of a toilet, and also made of porcelain. This bidet is situated right next to the toilet. Like a toilet they are permanently attached to the floor. Generally they need professional installation.

Classic Bidet A separate fixture like the toilet. Basically it is a large bowl that you can soak your buttocks in or squat over and splash yourself clean. Modern units have a dedicated water source: this one has a horizontal spray and a drain.

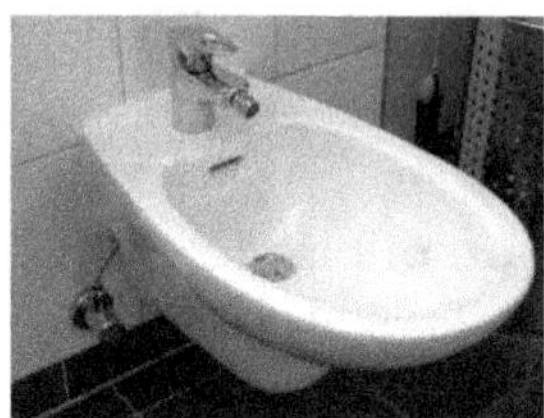

French Bidet The next evolutionary step. A separate fixture similar to the toilet, but definitely not a toilet, that has a water fountain or jet centered in the bottom of the bowl for washing your perianal area.

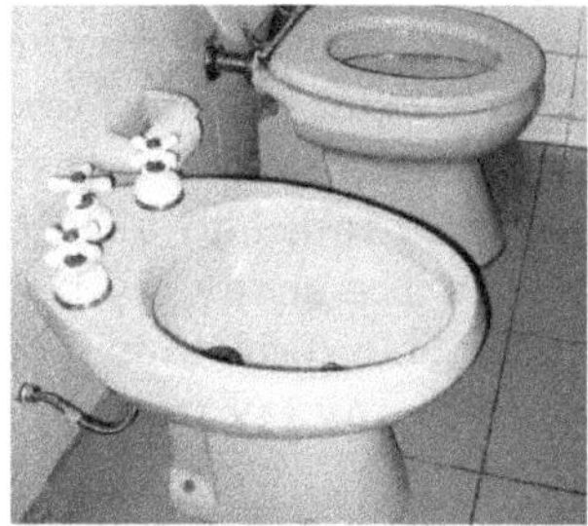

Clos O Mat The original integral bidet. A toilet with a built-in cleaning spray that fully cleans and then dries you. It has a number of conveniences for the severely disabled.

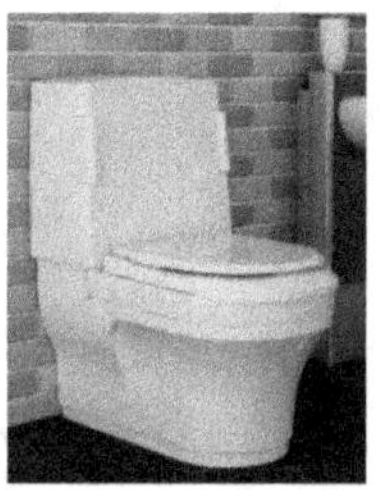
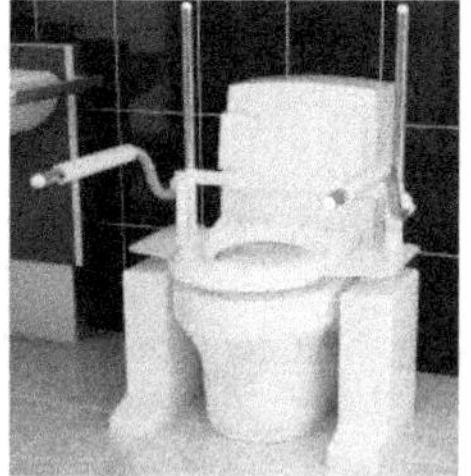

Mary Elizabeth Saga, who had a bidet installed in a new house she had built in Columbia, S.C., says she did have to explain what the bidet was to her builder: He said, 'Can you get me a picture of that or something.' I said, 'If you go to the plumbing supply store, they will tell you what a bidet is.' So he did and they told him that it was illegal because it was associated with houses of ill repute".[254]

Bidets Added To An Existing Toilet

TSB (Toilet seat bidet) Bidet plumbing that attaches to a toilet seat; bidet functions are integrated into a replacement toilet seat. Bidets almost always use the toilet's water supply. High-end units have all the physical functions of a shower toilet at a much lower cost. In addition there can be sophisticated integral electronics that can monitor your body's function from the toilet seat.[15]

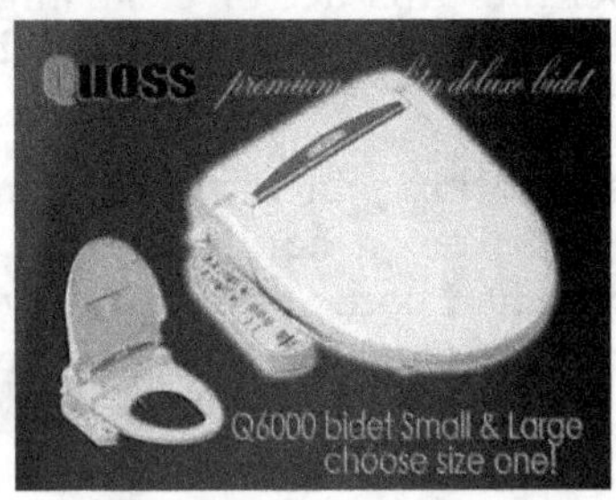

Hand-held bidet (Bidet Shower, Shattaf) Consists of a small flexible hose with a spray attachment that runs off of the water supply to the toilet. This can vary from vegetable sprayers designed for the kitchen sink, to "Shattaf" the ubiquitous hand sprayer of the Middle East, to advanced hand-held units with specialized sprays.

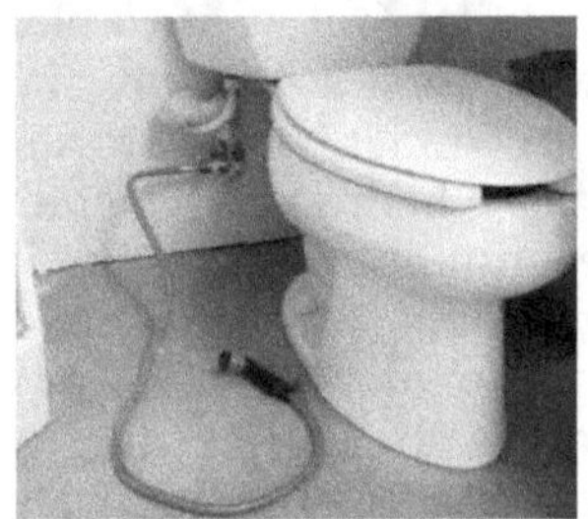

Bidets Separate From the Toilet

Travel bidet An independent hand-held spray unit with its own refillable water supply. It can be as simple as a squeeze bottle with a specialized tip or as complex as a battery-powered marvel with electronic adjustments.

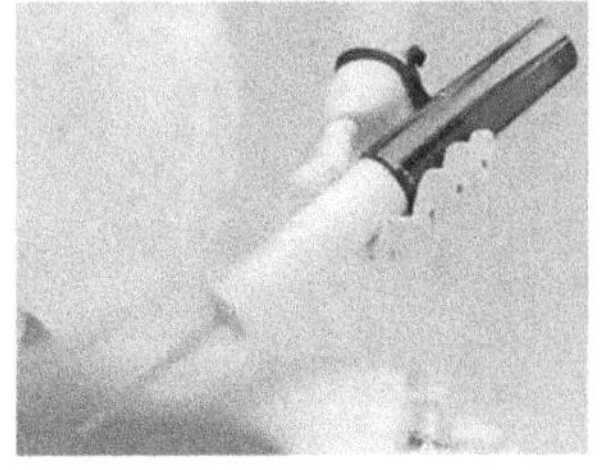

Bidet Floor Models

The (French) bidet started one of the most significant advances toward personal hygiene since the introduction of indoor plumbing. If it is logical to wash one's hands after going to the toilet, is it not even more fundamental to wash one's bottom? It is obviously impractical to take a tub or shower bath after every use of the toilet, but the bidet permits this act of cleansing by ablution without the necessity of disrobing. Therefore the bidet should be considered a hygienic necessity, rather than a luxury.[182]

In the 1980s a friend was working in Paris as contact person for a travel company. He received a call from a hotel after the departure of a group of Welsh rugby supporters who had come over for a Five Nations match. The girl at reception had wondered why some of them had edged down the stairs with their backs to the wall. All became clear when staff visited one of the rooms they had occupied. Apparently, they had removed the bidet and it must still sit somewhere as a trophy in a Welsh rugby club.[23]

The Classic Bidet

A classic bidet is a low mounted version of a sink or a shallow bath that was invented in the 17th century France, and ever since then used across the world as sanitation tool for washing legs, genitalia, inner buttocks and anus. Its name comes from the French world "bidet" which is translated as term "pony", but they also called it "trot", which is signifies someone riding a pony. They called it that way because of its use in the toilet (riding it to clean yourself), and sometimes bidet was even called "garden horse". Nobody today knows who exactly was responsible for the invention of bidet, but historians agree that they appeared first in 17th century France as a bedroom hygiene tool. From there it received several upgrades, until it eventually became an integral part of the modern bathroom. In the beginning, bidets were used in all French palaces and noble houses in the form of a traditional washbasin or a bathtub, only focused on washing feet and genitalia areas. In France they were regarded as a "civilized way" of preparing oneself for sex, or rinsing themselves after it.[53]

The original 18th century bidet was a portable sit-down wash basin into which water was poured for washing, and was not much more than a large pot. Traditionally the bowl was filled with water the same way you fill a tub - it essentially was a smaller version of a tub or sink - and subsequently was fitted with a stoppable drain for filling and emptying.[16-18] It operated much like a Sitz bath today. (See **Health**: Traditional Bidets and Sitz Baths).

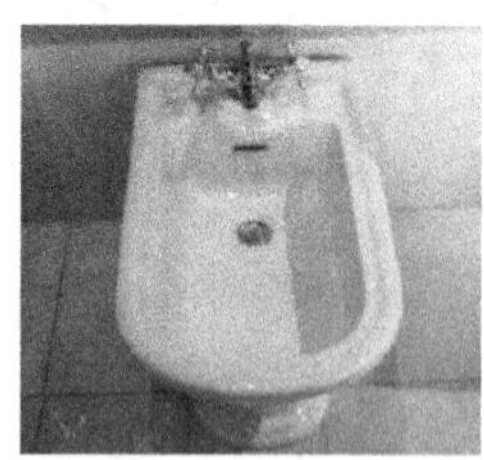

This classic bidet traditionally had no "toilet seat", and you straddled it backwards, facing the wall. I suppose that enabled one to be able to use water faucets if available, but have no idea why they would do this if a faucet wasn't available. It was traditionally styled to resemble the shape of the toilet. This classic style is still in use, with the addition of modern plumbing fixtures.[16-18]

The modern version is available in many designs and models, and is often offered as part of an integrated bathroom suite (like on this book's cover). Some models have a "toilet seat" and controls that allow you to sit forward as on a toilet. The bowl is still flooded, and needs no adjustment other than stopping up the drain and turning off the faucet if you do not want a constant flow of fresh water to drain away as you wash. Add a water jet and it becomes a French Bidet.

This bidet is permanently placed next to the toilet in the bathroom, allowing you to easily lateral from one unit to the other. The plumbing may have one tap (faucet) which pours cold water into the basin, or more likely two taps that allow you to adjust the water temperature. This bidet can also be equipped with a horizontal spray that can be useful for cleaning front to back when you face the wall.

This is generally the cheapest and simplest type of stand-alone bidet to install, though all the stand-alone bidets are more expensive than other bidets. This is due to two factors: the fixtures (taps, faucets, and spouts) are quite expensive, and any retrofit installation and plumbing of these units is both difficult and expensive. These separate bidets also take up significant space in the bathroom. This is offset by their simplicity of operation and the life-time durability after their installation. These days there are portable toilet inserts that function similarly as noted in the next section.

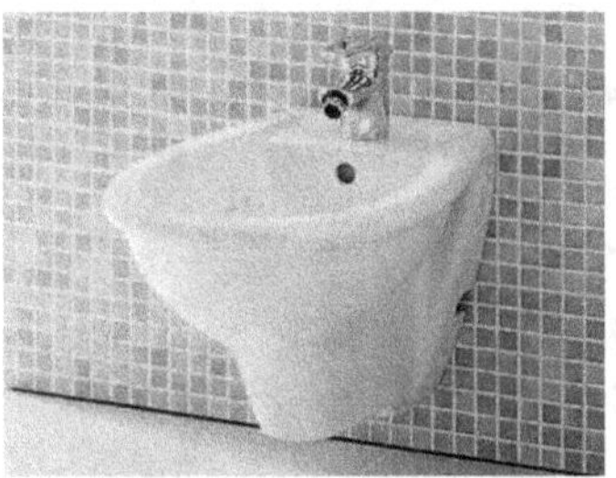

(It) comes in a variety of models, including both portable and wall mounted designs. Unlike the conventional sitz bath which forces patients to sit in their own contaminants, the unique flow-through design on the Hygenique Sitz Bath allows the user to drain contaminated water before the soothing warm water therapy begins. By combining a spray wand for bidet cleansing with a sitz bath for whirlpool heat therapy, (this) system provides a gentle and thorough cleansing which helps promote the healing process.... We primarily use (it) for rectal surgeries and some GYN procedures, and it has been very effective preventing infections with both. Nurse Manager[1]

When I was 14, we had our first family package holiday overseas to Calella in Spain and I saw a bidet for the first time. I had never seen one before and had no idea what it was for, but it was the ideal receptacle for washing my snorkel, mask and flippers after a hard days snorkelling in the Med.[23]

The French Bidet

Just ask Martina Rossi, lead singer of the band You Me and the Coffin. "When I've been traveling by myself or touring, staying at people's houses, I really, really missed it," she says. Martina is talking about my arch-nemesis, the bidet. "In Italy, where I live, it's just something that everybody has. It's like regular furniture in Italian people's houses," Martina says. "You have not much time and you can't take a shower, so it's just like, very fast and very useful".[73]

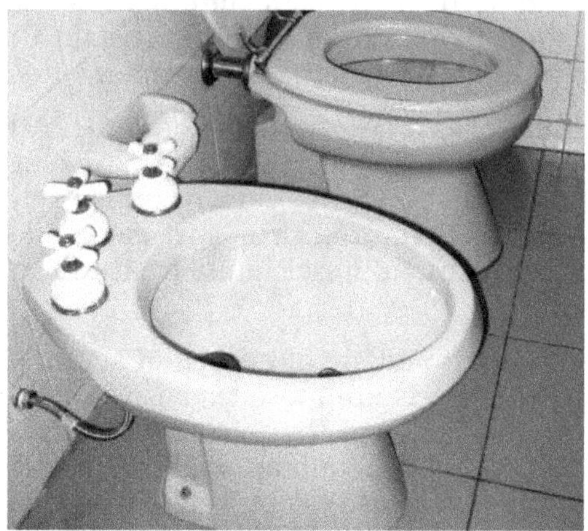

A 20th century standalone bidet

The first bidet that was more than a bowl on a stand was the bidet à seringue (syringe bidet) which was invented in 1750. It was operated with a hand-crank and produced a jet of water that was fed from a self-contained reservoir.[274] Modern plumbing and water pressure have transformed this into the classic French bidet, which turned what was a sit-down bath into a sit-down bottom shower.

The "French" bidet is a permanent, floor mounted plumbing fixture or type of sink intended for washing the genitalia, perineum, inner buttocks, and anus of the human body. It is usually located next to the toilet in the bathroom. One traditionally straddles it, facing the wall, with a water jet (fountain) in the center of the bowl.[16] There are many wry anecdotes on the Internet from travelers who incautiously turned on these bidets and washed the ceiling overhead, or got a face-full of water by bending over it.[12]

Similar to the classic bidet, you straddle this bidet and turn on the faucet. Which side you face is personal choice. Instead of filling the toilet bowl, a jet of water shoots up from the middle, washing your derriere clean. With a little movement you can position your genitals over this jet for additional cleaning. Other plumbing hardware offers jets that are adjustable for optimum washing.

Your germ-related comments are unfounded, since besides the vertical stream, there is a self-cleaning water function (bidets in Argentina have small holes in the rim pointing down and to the centre, delivering powerful streams of water on the basin surface in a way similar to a toilet flush).[12]

Here's the drill: Approach your bidet immediately after a bowel movement, bringing paper with you. I personally keep a roll of paper towels in the bathroom, as toilet paper disintegrates if used to dry your wet anus. Sit on the bidet FACING the controls, with your anus as low as possible in the bidet and just over the jets (you'll get the exact angle after a few tries, and no, at this angle used water does not wash down your legs--your anus is lower than your legs). A good bidet has cold and hot water faucets and a separate handle to activate the jet spray, just like a shower (like turning on the tub and then switching to the shower). If it matters to you, you can wait for the water to get warm before turning on the jet spray. Feel the jet spray hit your anus--it's very refreshing and some will use even more explicit adjectives of pleasure. I suggest assisting the cleaning process by reaching between your legs with your hand and using it to help clean (you'd do this in the shower, hopefully, so what's the difference, and you can wash your hands at the edge of the bidet after you turn off the spray). A little water splashed on your genitals AFTER cleaning your anus, is optional. After a vigorous cleaning use the paper towel to dry your anus (which should be so clean there's only water on the towel), discard the towel in the trash and wash your hands. You're fresh and clean, feel good, and have saved the water of a shower.[12]

It is important to note here that the above bidets were not meant to replace toilet paper, though they significantly reduce the amount used. The classic European routine is to defecate, wipe off with TP, and then move over to the bidet for final cleansing, and then dry yourself. I use a washcloth for drying which I change regularly. Usually it looks un-used when I wash it.

My friend's family who are "a bit posh" had one. As kids we figured out that the jet was so powerful it would just about reach the ceiling. So we had competitions to catch as much of the jet of water after it was coming back down from the ceiling in your mouth as you could. It wasn't easy. It was traveling fast and erratically and bounced out as soon as you tried to capture it. Mick, Northwood, UK[23]

There might be many times when you could use the bidet for a quick cleaning of your private parts without having defecated.[16] Bidets are also used for a variety of other cleaning tasks enumerated elsewhere. For examples see **Other Uses of The Bidet**.

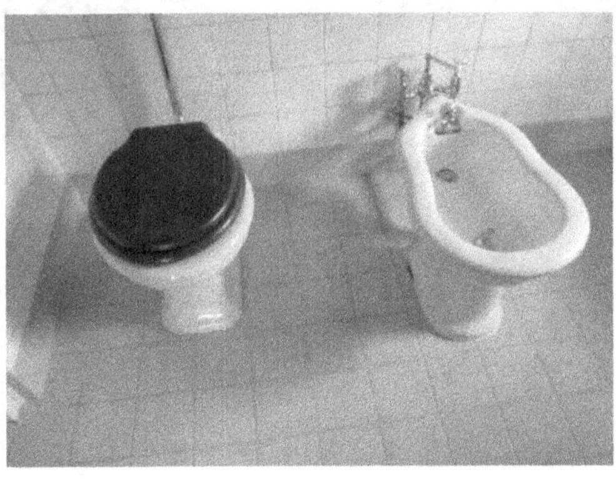

Clos-o-Mat (The Shower Toilet)

The next development in bidet design was immense, and happened in Switzerland in 1957. Hans Maurer invented the Clos-o-Mat, which combined a toilet with a bidet in the same unit. Basically a retractable bidet fountain was added with an air drier. This combined toilet and bidet was subsequently called a shower toilet. [13,24]

Maurer felt a genuine advance could be achieved only with the aid of a device which would make it possible to wash oneself immediately after the bowel evacuation, without previously wiping oneself dry. [24]

From the point of view of the bidet it was a revolutionary departure in design and function from the old eighteenth century model to one that was just then being embraced by modern society. Maurer felt "cleansing dirt from the body with dry paper" must be outdated by the mid 20th century and began designing equipment that would clean hygienically with warm water. [24]

Maurer's original invention came from a dream, but it was more like a nightmare for his first eight years of business, trying to create a useful and reliable product for a world that thought such a device was ridiculous and obscene. His stubbornness won out, creating rugged units known to provide over 20 years of reliable service, and slowly finding customers who were overjoyed with the results. It is amazing how one man's perseverance could eventually change how the world eliminates its personal wastes. [24]

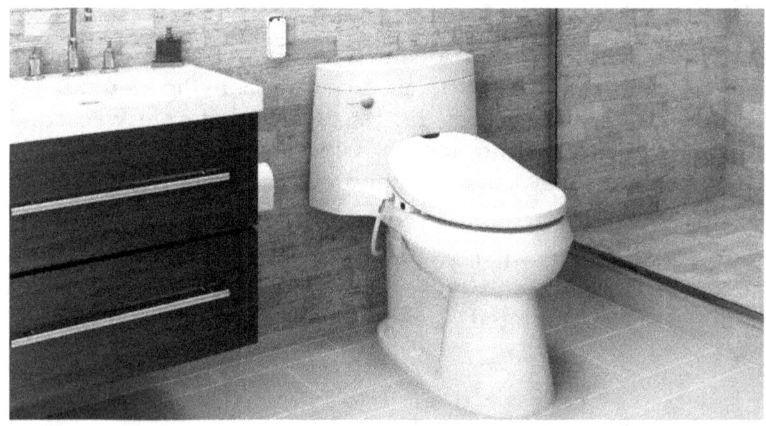

The Clos-O-Mat was the first device that combined the essential functions of wash, air dry, and deodorization, "that thoroughly services your hind quarters in a civilized fashion". The automatic nature of the device appeals to both the handicapped and able-bodied. Simply push a button and you are quickly finished - clean and dry. [25] The sticking point is that these units are very expensive: aside from the base cost, they must be plumbed in place like a toilet and have water and electrical connections made.

Neil Munro is a spokesman for the British supplier of these units. He tells me that in the United Kingdom the use of this type of product has largely been confined to "social needs" use (mainly to assist disabled people who cannot clean themselves) due to British Water bylaws. (Interesting - see Profound Ecology of the Bidet, for the fallacy of this.) He comments, "British culture is reluctant to accept the basic concept of cleansing by water after toileting – indeed I am sure you are aware personal hygiene toileting is almost regarded as a taboo subject in this country".[13]

Not to pick on the British, whom I find generally cleaner than us Americans, but the following study highlights the disconnect between perception and reality. Several sources cite a study of British men:

Paper cultures are in fact using the least efficient cleansing medium to clean the dirtiest part of their body. This point was memorably demonstrated by the valiant efforts of a Dr. J A Cameron, who in 1964 surveyed the underpants of 940 men of Oxford shire, England, and found fecal contamination in nearly all of them that ranged from a "wasp-colored" stains to "frank massive feces." Dr. Cameron, though a medical man, could not contain his dismay that "a high proportion of the population are prepared to cry aloud about footing matter of uncleanliness such as a tomato sauce stain on a restaurant tablecloth, while they luxuriate on a plush seat in their fecally stained pants.[8,123]

It is difficult, however, to suppress a smile at the irony of the situation. For years shit has been seen as something so repugnant that the word itself was scrubbed from polite conversation. The real reason for the ancient prejudice between urban and rural cultures was that before Fels-Naptha – the favorite heavy-duty farm soap – the odor of manure lingered on the skin and clothing of farmers. To become truly civilized mean to escape the barn and pretend that excrement was not a part of life – flush it and forget it. Even farmers bought into the notion. In 1961 Farm Journal, the leading farm magazine of the day, published an article arguing that manure was not worth hauling in the field. To its credit, the magazine renounced the error of its way in April of 1976 and rather lamely admitted that, in fact, manure was very much worth applying to cropland.... The larger animal factories today generate as much waste as the human sewage from a large metropolitan area, but, incredibly, they do not have to handle and treat their sewage the way municipalities do.[270]

While these floor models may be more than you can afford, read on. There are very functional bidets that fit any pocketbook. But first (next page) a humorous tale of a business exec's first encounter with an advanced Japanese bidet.

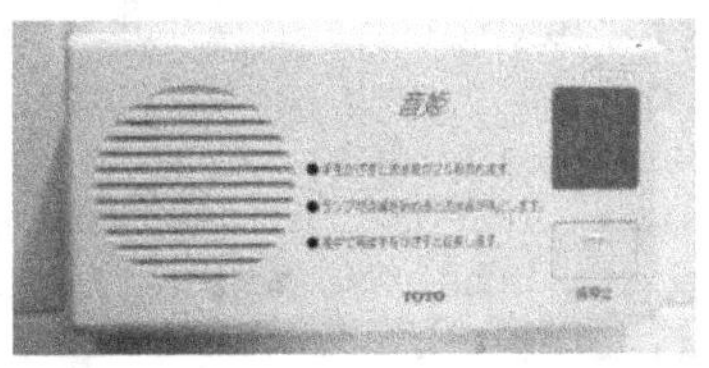

Modern Bidets

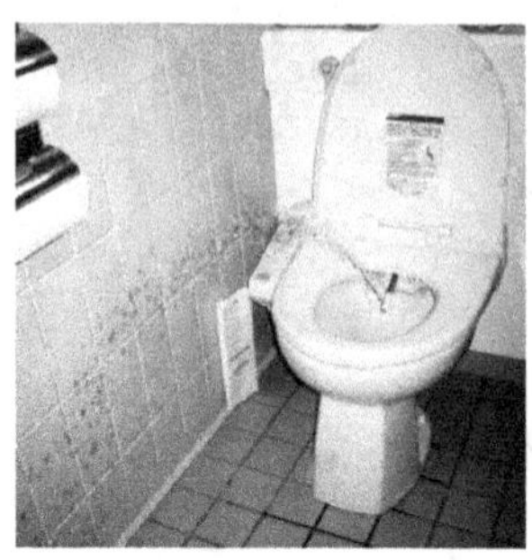

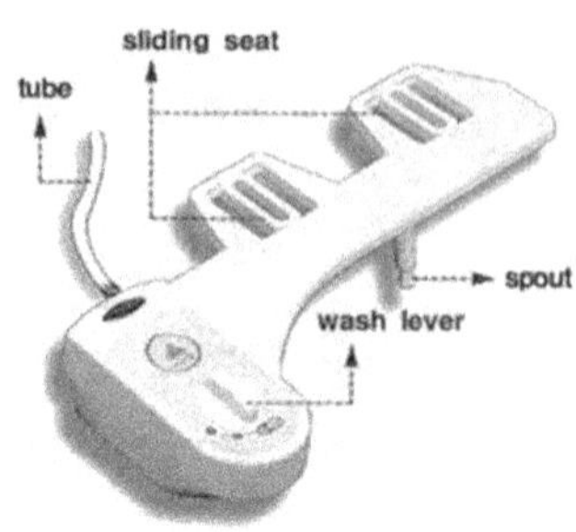

TSBs - Toilet Seat Bidets

First business trip to Japan 20 years ago. My hi-tech toilet in the hotel is connected to a huge panel full of buttons and controls, mounted on the opposite nearby wall, just within a stretch. No English. No cute little helpful icons. Only intimidating Japanese kangi, katakana, and hiragana characters. I didn't know it at the time, but that panel controlled water pressure, water volume, water temperature, angle of attack, and duration. Another set of buttons controlled the same things, except it was for the air-dryer. After staring incomprehensibly at the panel, I finally gave it a "oh what the hell" sigh and hit a random button. It was like I had activated an evil Rube Goldberg contraption that was to become the sentient forerunner of SkyNet.

The first fire hose blast up my anus required a fast desperate reaction, so I hit another random button. Bad, bad move. The fire hose started moving forward and blasted my balls like seriously-abused punching bags. While I'm madly scrambling for a third button, the punishing stream continued to move forward, contorting my snake into some kind of twisted art form and then finally up between my legs and into my face. During this assault, the water was steadily heating up to a definitely uncomfortable temp, and the hot blast to my face completely unnerved me. While grasping for the control panel, which I now could not see due to contact lenses being blasted into my brains, I fell forward off the toilet with my pants wrapped around my ankles, smacking my forehead on a small towel rack.

And there I lay, under a toilet shower, until everything finally cycled off—that is, after the interminable hissing of the air-dry cycle. I slowly and painfully crawled out of the bathroom on my stomach, bare buns-up, hoping that the toilet monster would not reawaken. My pants never fully dried before the next morning's business meeting, and the bruise above my left eye (and two blood-shot eyes) prompted my Japanese colleagues to jokingly remark what a wild night I must have had on the town.[84]

Best investment for the house. Originally I was going to buy the all in one toilet before I found out we could just buy the washlet without the toilet part. This saved us at least two thousand dollars but works just as great. Love the heated seating and temperature adjustment.[1]

These bidets attach to your toilet seat, or completely replace the toilet seat. Hans Maurer, inventor of the shower toilet, is reputed to also have developed the first toilet seat bidet -- the Clos-o-Mat Junior. Its production was discontinued due to significant technical and performance problems that could not be solved with 1960s technology. He did the best he could but it was twenty years too early.[13,24] The technology in bidets these days is completely digitized, fully functional and equipped with many comfort and convenience features for the user.

The "Classic TSB" is an all metal unit that attaches below the existing toilet seat with a lever that swings the bidet spray nozzle from the side into the middle of the toilet. The on/off valve also doubles as the flow control. Since these classic TSBs are not stand alone bidets, they generally only use "cold" water diverted from the toilet water supply. You have to move the lever around a bit, as well as moving your bottom around, to find the spots where the spray benefits you most. These are incredibly sturdy devices that last a lifetime, while providing the basic services of a bidet.

Times have changed. Mainstream TSB bidets now offer all the wonderful functionality of the original "shower toilet" with some modern technological additions at a fraction of the cost – truly affordable. Modern manufacturing and materials have helped develop TSB units that are sturdy and long-lasting, while exhibiting amazing functionality.

These new-age bidets will need a standard household electrical outlet to heat things up and to push air around.

Colorectal surgeons have been reluctant to use electronic bidets because the high force of water from commercially used electronic bidets may harm the anus.[20,106] On the other hand many users have eagerly embraced a more concentrated higher-pressure spray, when available, for the express purpose of inducing defecation.[130] All of this is fully adjustable with modern TSB bidets.

Mainstream bidets completely replace the toilet seat with a fully integrated unit that offers a wealth of basic options:

- Multiple adjustable nozzles
- Adjustable water pressure and temperature
- Independently create Warm/hot water
- Air drier,
- Air deodorizer,
- Self-cleaning nozzles,
- A heated toilet seat.

To put it bluntly: About one out of every seven trees we cut down goes straight into the toilet. But cultural biases and entrenched economics mean that the bidet is unlikely to save the world's forests; all signs point to continuing use of TP.[117]

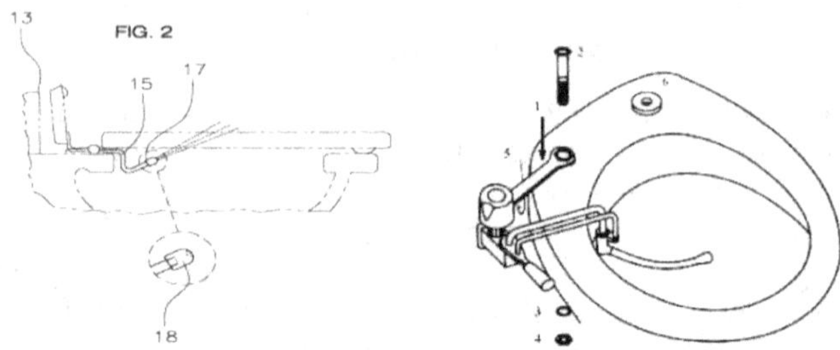

The most basic and primitive version of the TSB is simply a length of water tubing, an on/off valve that also acts as a crude water pressure control, and a small spray head attached to the end of the tubing. This unit takes water from the water line coming to the toilet and then snakes under the toilet seat and projects into the toilet bowl. A simple valve turns on the water. The cheapest TSB units may not even attach to the toilet seat, and depend on the stiffness of their piping to stay in place.

Slightly better TSBs have a plastic insert across the toilet bowl's back with a pressure activated nozzle. These TSBs are meant to stay in one position; they slide under the toilet seat and remain in that position except for cleaning. A pressure-activated nozzle protrudes into the toilet bowl a few inches. The non-adjustable spray head extends to just before and below where you defecate. After you perform your act of elimination, you turn it on and a spray of water is directed at your anus and genitals.

While a simple unit like this can provide the basic service of washing your bottom clean, it has several drawbacks. First, it is fixed into one position that may not be appropriate for everyone using that toilet, or even appropriate for both anal and genital washing of one person.

Second, because it is always in position, and must always be safely behind where everyone defecates, the spray often is directed up and forward. I personally have found this unhealthy, because the feces are washed towards the genitals and I found myself having skin problems around my genitalia. (More in **Health Benefits** - Infection.) It is possible that this may not be a problem for you.

Best seat in the house! My wife and kids thought I was crazy when I was finishing our walk-out basement and wired electrical right by the toilet location because I told them I was putting in "The Greatest Toilet Ever". They now understand. The kids love the heated seat. I love the reduction in toilet paper usage. I need to put three more in now.[1]

Immediately after surgery I regretted not following up on my thoughts to get a bidet. With the dry or even wet wipes causing pain, burning and great irritation to my incisions washing by hand was the only option for weeks. I must say they were right on, it's just fantastic. No more incision BURN and irritation and now I am able to clean deep inside the rectum effortlesy and most importantly, hands free - this system is just fantastic, absolutely FANTASTIC![1]

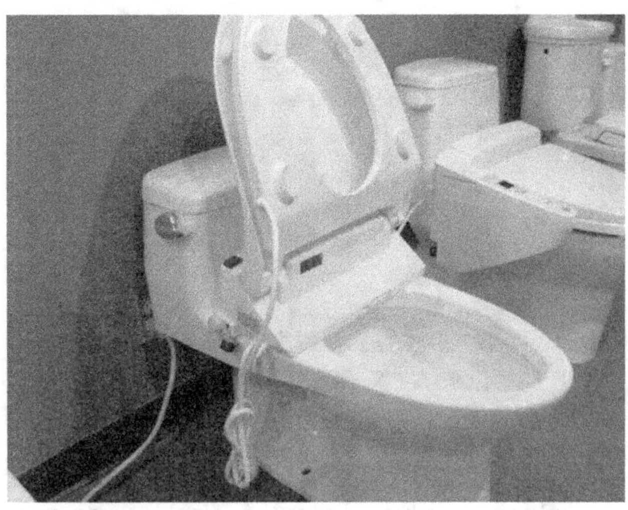

The next step up are TSBs that have one or more pressure activated arms with spray heads that extend further and adjust to your best angles. A basic unit has the classic vertical spray which seems to suit most users. More advanced models allow multiple spray heads, angles and patterns to suit your every need. A spray head extends out only when needed. Many now have remote controls, some remember your preferred settings, and most have some sort of self-cleaning.

One simple refinement is the addition of a hot water supply so that you can set the water temperature, which is adjustable to a user's individual preferences. The warmed water typically comes from an on-demand water heater built-in to the toilet seat. This requires an electrical connection.

There are some units that pipe in the hot water from the sink, which has the advantages of being quite reliable and independent of electricity. The disadvantages of these models are even more visible piping and a much slower warm-up of the water.

Modern technology and materials have eliminated the need for a "separate toilet" taking up precious space in the bathroom. Complete bidet packages are easily attached to your existing toilet as a replacement toilet seat, and there is an effective bidet for nearly every pocketbook.[13]

Wonderful. Discovered these in Japan and boy are they wonderful. Bought one for the bedroom and it works fantastic. You feel so clean after using the Washlet. This model allows you to determine warmth level for the wash, the seat, and the dryer. Yes, it has a blow dryer. You can also adjust the water pressure. You can use a button to wash the gadget that washes you. Also, as soon as you sit, water is sprayed around the inside of the toilet so nothing "sticks" to it, which is very nice. And the whole thing is very quiet. For the price I was very impressed with the feature and how well it works.[1]

Advanced TSBs

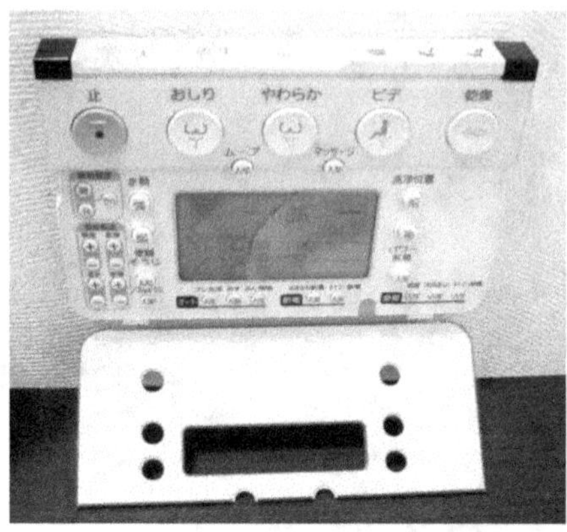

You feel so much cleaner.... I found out about these Washlets on a trip to Japan where they are almost everywhere. I visited a Buddhist monastery up on a mountain and the solitary monk said that the Washlet was one of the reasons he like that particular place.... I have other toilets in my house, but I never use them. It's worth the walk to go to the Toto. It may sound frivolous, but you just have to try this.[1]

The more advanced TSBs offer stainless steel self-cleaning nozzles, adjustable nozzle position, adjustable pressure, adjustable water temperature, remote control, heated bidet seat, heated air dryer, and effective deodorizers. You typically have a choice of sprays: the standard is one or more vertical fountain jets from the center of the bowl, plus an angled stream of water intended to protect the genitalia. The sprays are all configured with different pressures, patterns, air/water cleansing, and "touch" appropriate for their function.

Models currently on the market have fans that "break down odorous molecules," digital clocks to tell users how long they have been on the toilet, a control panel that offers a choice of flush strengths, and devices that automatically put the seat down when you are done... The idea of the high-tech toilets, one researcher told the Washington Post is to make the bathroom a place where people can relax.[184]

Bidet air deodorizers use a fan to increase the air that circulates, and this means more air is cleaned and deodorized. The fan pulls in air that has odors and removes the particles with the carbon filtration system in the toilet seat, and this is very effective at truly deodorizing rather than simply covering up the odors in your bathroom... Through the process of adsorption the bidet deodorizers remove the unpleasant smells from the air.[87]

With top-of-the-Line TSBs everything is fastidiously cleaned. It can anticipate your (or anyone's) patterns of need. You have complete control over when and how it starts, water temperature, water pressure, seat warming, air drying, and odor elimination. Multiple spray attachments extend and withdraw. Health monitoring is an increasing function, and units are increasingly connected to the internet.

Toto is working on smart toilets that measure "input" and "output" and send the information to health care services. These toilets talk to their users, take their weight and blood pressure, measure body fat using electric currents, measure chemicals in the urine to determine glucose levels and, someday, cancer, and send results online to medical facilities. These toilets are being offered for $4,000 in new houses built by Daiwa house. Some new toilets have ejector-seat like contraptions that help elderly people and handicapped people get off the seats... Toto's newest Neorest systems have wall control panels, stereos, buttons that adjust water pressure and air purification. There are also modals that offer massages with gentle pulses of water and anticipate the approach of users with sensing devices and open the lid automatically so you don't have to touch anything. These units send out "etiquette" music of river and bird sounds and employ deodorizers that use activated oxygen to remove odors at the molecular level and release rose and cherry blossom fragrances. Among those who have purchased them are the actor Will Smith.[184]

Toto in Japan will sell you a floor model of its advanced bidets, but their TSBs offer the same features. The plumbing setup for a floor model is more expensive, more complex and can be more unsightly, if it ends up external to the unit.

The other plus of a floor model is that they are insanely durable and trouble-free. Wear and tear on TSBs is bound to be more of an issue, though vendors of these top-line units generally can't remember when a unit was returned for repairs.

With TSBs you are only limited by your budget and your own personal preferences. Once you start looking at bidet toilet seats and comparing various manufacturers and models you are sure to find some that fit your budget and your needs.

If you got something full of germs and bacteria on your hands or arms you wouldn't just wipe it with a paper towel until it came back clean would you? You wouldn't feel like you got your hands clean unless you scrubbed with soap and water! You would use at least water to clean it off so why only use dry toilet paper on your bottom? It is a sensitive area that you should treat as best as you could to maintain the best hygiene and prevent future problems and toilet paper alone is not the best you can do.[28]

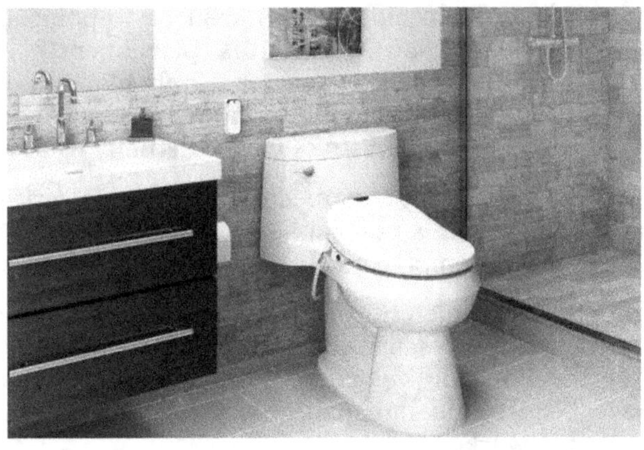

Handheld & Portable Bidets

The last time I went to Korea was in 2006 and almost every home bathroom had a bidet with a little remote at the side to choose different functions like spray my butthole, clean the bowl, blow my butt with warm air. That shit was glorious.... What about the handheld sprayer kinds? Those are honestly my fav from traveling around, and I would think any one you get would be BIFL. It's just a steel hose and sprayer, like you find on most kitchen sinks nowadays.[246]

I went to Thailand and the bathrooms there are terrible- but they have AWESOME bum guns! - Evan S., America/Mexico.[274]

"I normally don't do testimonials, but I feel so strong about this product that I have a hard time keeping my mouth shut. Had two hip replacements last year, really came in handy. I liked it so much I put it on my 40 ft. boat. No more clogged heads. Once you use it you will never go back to paper. I think I will give one to my Mom who is in an assisted living home. Try it you will like it."[41]

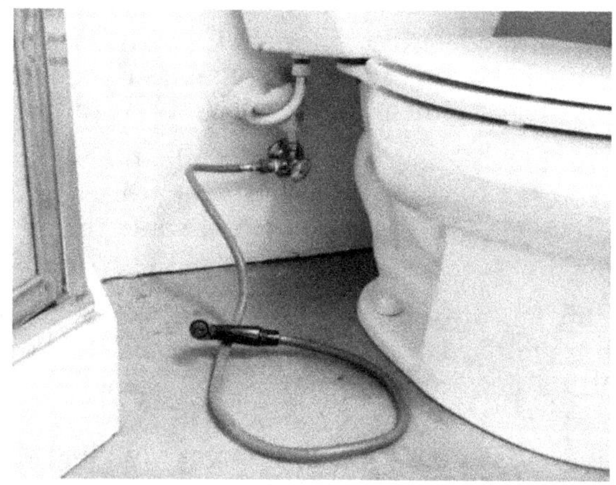

Note the drying rag tucked under the toilet water reservoir

There are two types of handheld bidets, both are free to point and spray in any direction you choose (good and bad). The first is "permanently" connected to the toilet system, and taps into to the toilet's water supply like other bidets, but on a flexible hose. It must be held in the hand and aimed to be used. It is not unlike the vegetable sprayer on your kitchen sink (That is actually what I use).

This is accomplished by adding a "T-connector" to the pipe carrying water to the toilet. This usually only requires some pliers, and can thus easily removed if needed. Some renters will assemble and cleanly disassemble when they leave.

Another type of bidet is a completely portable unit. It can be a fancy model that is battery powered and pump-pressurized, or it can be as simple as a specially-shaped squeeze bottle. Portable bidets all have their own water supply. These types of units have been found indispensable for travelers, both business and pleasure, and homecare workers.

Handheld Bidet Attached To The Toilet

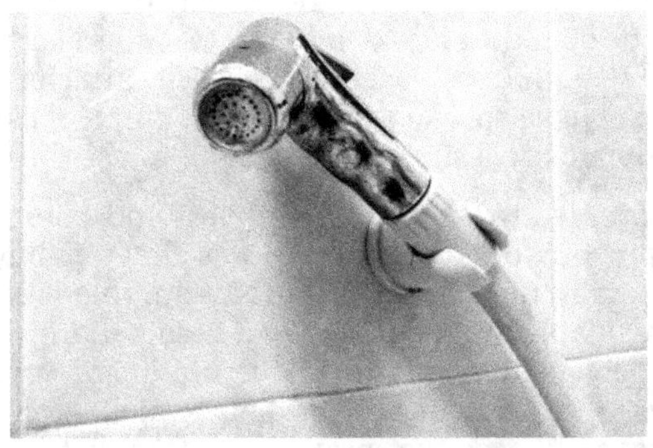

Travelers tell me that hand sprayers are often found as adjuncts in bathrooms throughout Europe, the Middle East (the Muslim Shattaf), and Asia, partly for personal hygiene, but also for general bathroom clean-up and for such tasks as washing out diapers. There is not a lot of difference between hand sprayers. Nearly all use cold water only – although there are warm water units which use additional piping and attach to the sink spigots.[19] Most people actually prefer the cold water units. Generally, the choices are mostly design and styling but the choice of spray head can be significant. An important factor would be jet design - how many and how they are arranged.

If you are poor (or cheap) these are your bidets. The commercial units can be as cheap as $25 delivered, and include everything you need to set them up. These units come with full hardware and instructions, and generally need only a screwdriver and pliers (or worst case wrench) as tools.

Believe me, ye of little faith, a bidet, or whatever name you would give to an anal cleansing pistol/device, is a f****** godsend. I lived in SE Asia for a bit, and once you get used to one of these things (mine was the handheld version, a stand-alone anal water pistol which hung on the wall next to the toilet), there's no going back. Westerners use toilet paper to smear shit all over their arses, and consider themselves "clean" when the paper comes back more-or-less unbrowned. Horseshit! Use one of these and a quick check using TP will tell you that bun blasting is the only way to truly clean your nether regions.[12]

My bidet for the past sixteen years has been an inexpensive vegetable sprayer often found as part of the kitchen sink. Why? While building my new house I had designed in a floor model bidet to be part of the bathroom, but last minute changes in the plans left me without the room to install it. It also offended my Scottish bones that, while a whole new toilet costs only about $150; floor bidets (structurally the same) start around $600 plus installation.

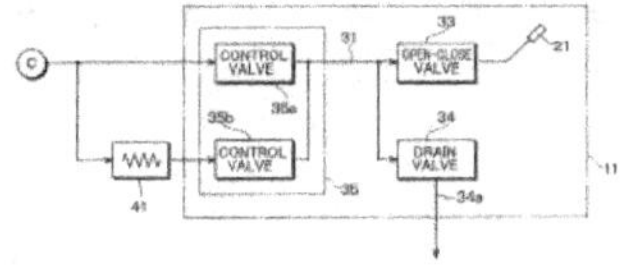

Yet, I really, really wanted the benefits of a bidet. While installing the kitchen sink I noticed the vegetable sprayer attachment and thought, "This could work!" This was before I was aware that there are handheld sprayers all over the world that are specifically designed to act as a bidet. Commercial bidet units start out slightly more expensive than a vegetable sprayer attachment, and are more ruggedly built and may have special spray heads. Complete assembly instructions and attachment hardware are a strong inducement to use the commercial units.

You would be hard pressed to find a more modest and minimal "bidet" than the one I use, yet this sprayer works well for me, was cheap to buy and install, and is easy to replace. Generally these units are pretty durable. My first unit was very cheap, even for a vegetable sprayer, and as a result didn't spray very well and within months stopped up with grit from our unfiltered spring water system. I then bought the best replacement spray heads available at the hardware store (still under $10). I have replaced the spray head probably three times in 16 years.

It is good to have one of these handhelds around even if you own another type of bidet. I would not replace mine with a TSB unit until I could afford a high-end model with the seat warmer, warmer water and air-dry features.

A huge bonus is this type of unit's availability for other cleaning tasks. I can do a light cleaning of the toilet bowl. The spray at full strength can actually clear a mild blockage of the toilet, if you still have blockages once you stop using toilet paper. My unit can just reach into the shower stall for cleaning there as well. Read more in **Other Uses of The Bidet** for more on this.

In the USA alone around 36.5 billion rolls of toilet paper are used every year, and this can have an enormous cost in terms of energy use. The manufacturing process for this amount of toilet paper will require approximately 17 terawatts of electricity each year, including the packaging and transportation of the finished rolls. Recycling one single ton of paper can save over 4,000 kilowatt hours of energy, and this amount can power the average home in America for 6 months as well as saving 17 trees from being cut down.[87]

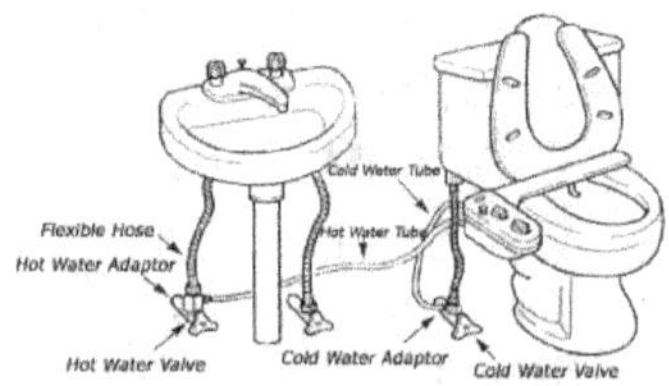

I think in Asia, the bidets there are more like the bidet sprays, which are attached to the toilet, unlike the European versions which is a different toilet altogether. I did get one like the Asian style. At first it was really uncomfortable, but I got used to it. Can't use that for washing feet or babies or chilling beer though haha![216]

Portable Bidets

These portable bidets are actually in a category of their own, since they alone are not attached to the toilet at all. They are self-contained (they have their own water supply rather than using the existing plumbing like the other bidets). There are two iterations of this device: powered and hand-squeeze.

For someone with hemorrhoids and allergies to preservatives (like benzalkonium chloride) in some wet wipes and witch hazel pads, I gave this device a try. There is a very short period of adjustment where you need to learn how to aim the device, but after 2-3 tries your placement of the spray will be fine. It does make some noise (like an electric toothbrush or carving knife) so there would be no possibility to use it discretely in a public washroom -- unless you really didn't care. This is much gentler on inflamed tissues and does a good job of cleaning the nooks and crannies you can't even see. I do use it a couple times just to be sure everything is flushed away, followed by dabbing with tissues and drying with warm air. Then, any creams could be applied, if needed. I believe it has helped considerably and I'm glad I purchased it.[1]

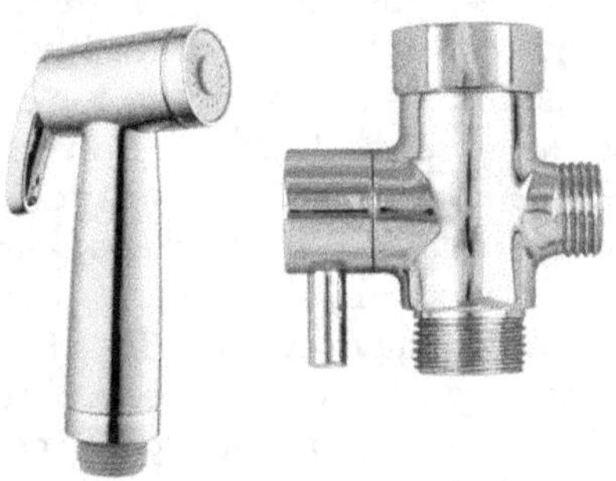

Pressure Powered Portable Bidets

A portable bidet can run on battery power, or can be physically pressurized with a hand pump. This self-contained-ness and independence is very attractive to travelers who may find themselves in places with primitive or "iffy" facilities.

I was surprised that travel bidets are a lot more varied and sophisticated than standard hand-held units. Travel is a flexible term - I suspect that a lot of these units go to the office every day, or reside in the glove compartment of many cars. They are inexpensive enough to be very cheap insurance for some of life's disastrous or difficult moments.

"As we started on a three week trek through India, my friends roared with laughter when they heard about my Travel Washlet. But by the end of the trip, they were jealous and asked to borrow it. I used it forty to fifty times; it performed flawlessly and still has its original battery. Congratulations on a terrific product!" Dr. A. Cohen.[124]

However, over that period standard toilet paper rolls accounted for only 1.3 billion rolls to this growth. In 1981 Georgia Pacific launched a new premium quality "thick, strong and soft" toilet paper brand - Moltonel - and over the course of the subsequent two and a helf decades this new premium "thick, strong and soft" segment came to account for a quarter of the total category growth adding 300 million rolls to annual consumption.[244]

The limitations of the battery-powered units are: (1) batteries may limit the water pressure "punch" available, (2) battery life is always an issue, though these units seem to be quite frugal on electricity, and (3) small water reservoirs limit washing time.

They make up for this with technology. Efficient, powerful low-voltage pumps with easily interchangeable jets can provide significant adaptability to your needs. They offer pulsing streams of water for maximum cleaning. Some jets oscillate, making the process more automatic, perhaps also with air bubbles to enhance cleansing. These units have the additional advantage of using either warm or cold water, as well as the option of adding cleaning agents to the small water tank.

I've just returned from a three week trip in Europe. I used this device daily. It's compact, light, solid, and works so well I'd use it for home daily use if I didn't have a Toto seat top washlet. It's spray is fine for cleaning me, and it doesn't get soiled in use, though I give it a light soap down and rinse every time just in case. Very little effort is needed to set it up and fill with water, use, and re-pack. One battery lasted 15 days of regular use, and then I replaced it just in case. The specs indicate 50 hours of run time per battery, but that seems impossible. However, I could have left the first battery in just to see. For a month's trip for one person I'd recommend one spare AA alkaline battery, and no more. The storage bag has a tough plastic opener for the battery cover, so no coins are ever needed to unscrew the cap, which is sealed and waterproofed, as is the whole unit. Toilet paper just isn't needed, except for maybe a little pat down to dry yourself after cleaning. Much of the world beyond the nice hotels can't deal with toilet paper in the sewer system, and this is the solution to that problem. I tended to use one refill per use, and a water bottle makes that simple. Its noise is too minor for concern unless you're really, really shy. If toilet paper is a pain for you to use, then just buy this thing.[1]

The Toto travel Washlet is, in fact, nothing more than a water pick for your butt. The real proof, however, is in the "last swipe" of toilet tissue: the "white glove test," if you will. I begrudgingly admit that this automatic, battery-operated bidet works very, very well — again, perhaps not 70-something-dollars better than the cheapest alternative, but certainly well enough. It's definitely "nice-to-have", a creature-comfort.[1]

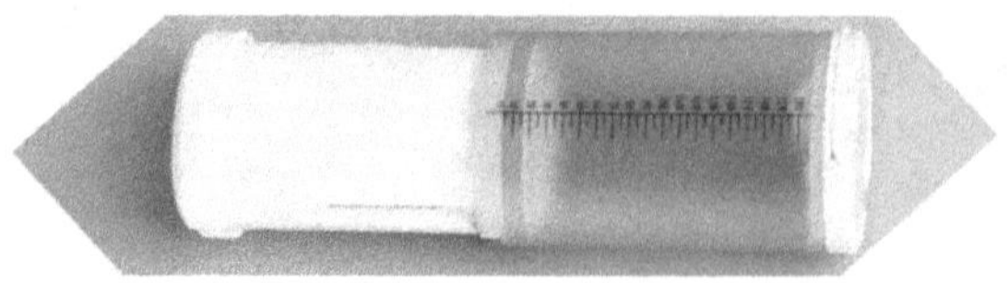

Squeeze-Bottle Portable Bidet

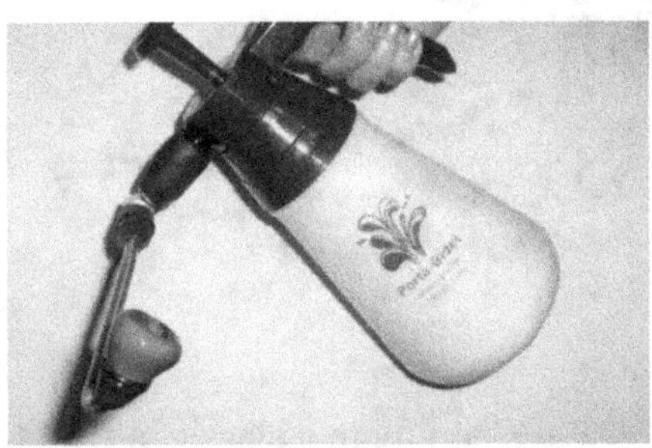

Talk about primitive tech! Pretty much any squeezable plastic bottle with any sort of nozzle cap can be a portable bidet, but a specially shaped bottle top is what you would be buying. For example a dedicated nasal wash squeeze-bottle could work and are easily available. Bidet bottles with a specially designed cap can deliver a good cleaning spray for the anus and the perianal region.

There is a learning curve when using all hand-held units. Do not use one for the first time in the executive washroom! Learning how to use a traveler's hand-held unit out on the trail is an attractive notion, as learning with these units at the outset can be messy. Read more about this in **Cleaning With A Bidet**.

A growth area for portable bidets is traveling healthcare providers. These units have been shown to make the life of visiting healthcare workers much easier.[267]

It was a hit with my wife and her girlfriends at the camping site. The children want to use it for squirt gun so be prepared for that.[1]

This product is amazing! I took it with me to Burning Man since it's a serious porta-potty situation and you cannot throw even flushable wipes into them - TP only. So this little gem worked like a charm! Everyone I showed it to was amazed and many of them will be ordering one for next year's Burn. There are two settings for the water stream force you want and it amazingly runs on 1 battery. It's light, easy to travel with, and was a lifesaver. This made my experience so much better and I would definitely recommend this product. In fact, I already have and it was quite the buzz in my camp![1]

Outstanding product for the price. After only a couple months using it, going on vacation and using a hotel bathroom without one felt barbaric, like squatting in the woods and wiping with pine needles. It works as advertised! Truly it is the bidet that separates us from the animals. John B [248]

A hand held bathroom bidet sprayer is so much better than a stand alone bidet and this is why:1.It's less expensive (potentially allot less) 2.You can install in yourself = no plumber expense 3.It works better by providing more control of where the water spray goes and a greater volume of water flow. 4.It requires no electricity and there are few things that can go wrong with it. 5.It doesn't take up any more space, many bathrooms don't have room for a stand alone bidet. 6.You don't have to get up and move from the toilet to the bidet which can be rather awkward at times to say the least.[311]

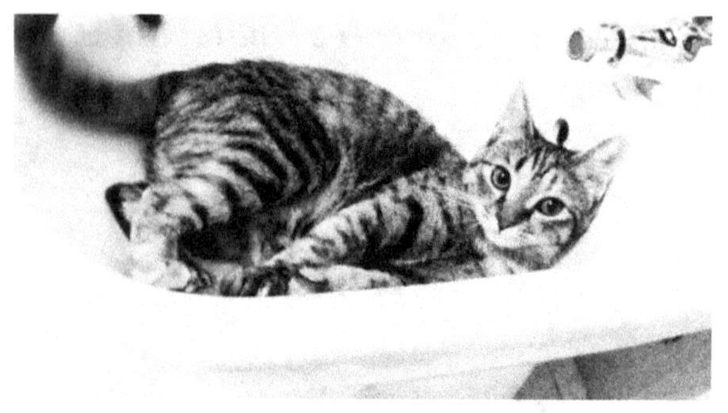

Cat sleeping in a classic bidet

Benefits Of The Bidet

Who benefits from using the bidet? Anyone. Everyone. There are multiple benefits for anyone who uses a bidet, some of which have already been noted. Everyone with special needs have already found that bidets offer them significant and crucial personal service. Here we will more clearly delineate all the benefits that bidets can offer. This section will discuss two main categories of benefit: Cleanliness and Health, with the profound ecology of the bidet overall.

Bidet Cleanliness

So are Americans the world's cleanest people? They scent their toilet-paper and decorate it with flowers, but unlike the Japanese they are not "a people who like to wash their bottoms" and neither the French bidet nor the Japanese Toto toilet finds many customers in the United States. We think talking cleanliness so far is dirty.[6]

Toilet paper is not hygienic at all. It's the equivalent of cleaning your dishes by wiping them with a dry piece of paper and then putting them back in the cabinet.[216]

It has been estimated that there are some 12 million persons in the United States who suffer from arthritis and rheumatism, some 2 million hemiplegic (stroke) victims, 500,000 who suffer from Parkinson's disease, 100,000 paraplegics and quadriplegics, 200,000 who suffer from muscular dystrophy, 500,000 with multiple sclerosis, and 500,000 victims of cerebral palsy. In a substantial number of instances, these are the people likely to suffer the most severe impairment of their locomotor activities - and hence their ability to manage with conventional hygiene accommodations.[8]

We are an obstetrics and gynecology office and it works very well for our patients' needs. Dr. Laura Goldstein East Side Women's Ob/Gyn Assoc.[124]

We are a prenatal clinic and birthing center. Our clients seem to like the washlets a lot! Elizabeth Seton Childbearing Center, New York City[124]

The psychological, as well as the physical, problems associated with personal hygiene are vastly more complex and difficult for persons with disabilities and handicaps than for others, and it needs to be recognized that they are as difficult for the person directly involved as for persons associated with them.... For the benefit of the sceptics or the guilt-ridden, note that the sensation resulting from our common habit of dry-wiping - once one has become accustomed to washing - has been compared by some to the sensation resulting from not brushing one's teeth from one week to the next.[8]

The most important form of non-medical management is to improve hygiene to ensure that the perianal area is cleansed of fecal deposits or urine, that irritate the skin, in a way that does not further irritate the skin (e.g. by excessive rubbing or exposure to harsh soaps and detergents or allergens). Instead, bidets (or baths), soft wet washcloths (or cotton balls) or unscented baby wipes are recommended.[237]

The therapeutic advantages of washing after elimination, as well as the benefits of increased cleanliness in the perineal area, should be obvious to every proctologist, gynecologist and general physician. Bathing the perianal area and genital organs can be more easily and frequently accomplished with a bidet than in a tub or shower. Women should thoroughly cleanse their external vaginal area at every opportunity during their menstruation period.

My husband and I are both medical professionals and we are happy to endorse the TOTO Washlet. We have a Washlet S300 (Jasmin) in our home and a Travel Washlet for travel. We feel that your products have brought personal hygiene into the twenty-first century, and that no home should be without them. Donna M. Guttman, R.N.& Donald I. Guttman, M.D. [124]

I have a friend whose rear end is very sensitive, and chronically inflamed from wiping with toilet paper. He always has to buy those moistened, medicated wipes, yet still lingers on the edge of despair, due to the film (or coating) of feces inevitably left by wiping. Some of his most sensitive skin is almost perpetually coated with dangerous bacteria, as is anyone using toilet paper.

Then consider his alternative - always being clean. He can clean himself with very accurate localized washing, while stimulating his immune system and soothing his chafed skin with hydro-massage one or more times daily. He can do this without having to undress, take a complete shower, or towel off. Many units can air-dry his skin. Others allow him to add soap, disinfectants, or anything else to the water supply should he need them. Clean water itself is wonderfully therapeutic[37], and with the chlorine in most water supplies, is also mildly antiseptic. Imagine feeling shower clean after a bowel movement!

Caveat: Pure cold water is least irritating to the skin. As water gets hotter, it gets slightly more irritating. Chlorine does irritate. Soap and water, however beneficial, are more irritating still. Too many washings a day with soap and warm water can chafe the skin.[29-33] Read more about water in **Water and the Bidet**.

Elderly and Physically Challenged

Our Institute has investigated the expressed needs of many severely disabled people. One requirement was for a portable bidet that would fit on a standard toilet, so that they could still have some of the advantages of their automatic washing/drying/flushing toilet when away from their own house.... It allows a user with very weak arms to wash themselves with warm water, and a hands-free drying method is explained in the instruction booklet.... (and) can be controlled by commercially available single switch activators, so that any user can operate it.[26]

A little old man who's hard of hearing goes to see the doctor. As he can't hear very well, he takes his wife with him. The doctor examines the man and then says, "Hmm, I think we need to take a stool sample, a urine sample and a sperm sample." The old man turns to his wife and asks, "What did he say?" The wife replies, "He said he wants your underwear".[298]

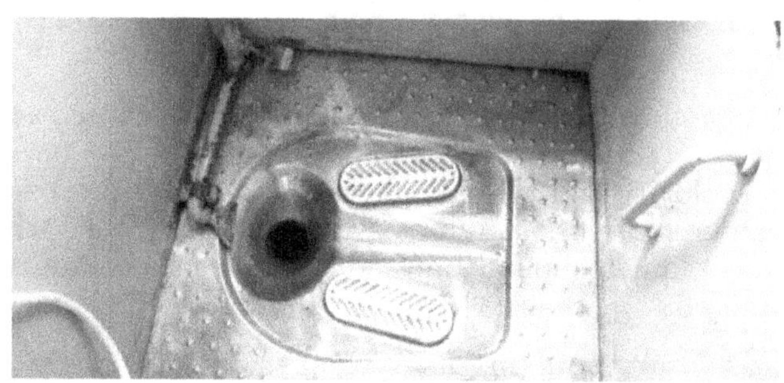

Elderly people and persons with a disability may face significant limitations when using the standard "sitting" type water toilet as mostly used in the Western World. In this paper a new type of a stationary robotic toilet is outlined and the concept of the smart interaction between user and envisaged robotic toilet is described. Main functionality are height and tilt adjustment, support of sitting down and standing up, speech interaction, automatic recognition of the user and corresponding preferred settings of the toilet and automatic inference of potential emergency situations. The interaction is challenging due to the very different needs of the target group, the physical contact to the robotic system (actually the user is sitting on the robot) and the taboo area of toileting.[229]

I give it five stars and my only regret is I didn't get one earlier...Having suffered lower spinal problems, twisting and turning has made my life problematic in regards to personal hygiene in the bathroom! This bidet has been the best thing that has ever happened! I give it five stars and my only regret is I didn't get one earlier, life is so much less frustrating since it has been installed! Sincerely, A Delighted Customer.[41]

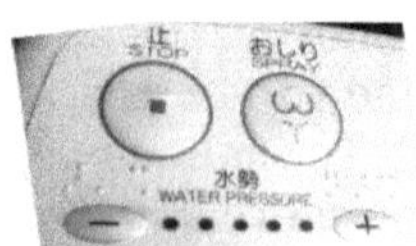

This has been a growth niche for bidets. Senior citizens often have physical limitations, as do those who are disabled, incontinent, in chronic pain, or mentally challenged. Others find standing, reaching, bending, and other movements are painful, difficult, or impossible to accomplish. All of these individuals can benefit greatly from using some form of bidet. Many different designs exist and combined toilet-bidets are proving popular in the elderly population.

We invented Perijett at the request of a disabled military veteran who had to rely on someone to assist him when he needed to toilet. His added challenges included incontinence. Our flagship product, the Perijett, exceeds the capabilities of the standard toilet seat bidet. In addition to a gentle water rinse Perijett offers the ability to administer a topical OTC perineal wash upon demand. The Perijett is an FDA classified Class 1 exempt perineal care device manufactured in the U.S.A. The Perijett has also proved to be an essential hygienic fixture for (i) those with a limited range of motion due to arm, hip, or back surgery - especially rotator cuff surgery, (ii) elderly and bariatric patients, (iii) anyone needing a raised toilet seat, (iv) incontinence. We recently received a GSA contract award (#36F79718D0483) to provide Perijett hygiene assist devices to VA.[41]

Specifically, people with impaired motor functions (mild or moderate Alzheimer's disease, cerebral palsy, arthritis, muscular dystrophy, or multiple sclerosis, for example) have a humiliating limitation on their ability to wipe themselves off after using the toilet. Severely overweight people often have these limitations as well. Those bidets that are combined with the toilet provide simple, one-handed controls to thoroughly cleanse after elimination, and better models will dry you as well.[34-7]

My hubby's had a bidet for years. He has back trouble, and the bidet made life easier. But I'm fat, and his bidet wasn't a good fit for me. I tried the Bio Bidet TP-70 Travel Bidet with Extended Nozzle, Brondell GS-70 GoSpa Travel Bidet Travel Bidet, and the Giraf Portable Travel Bidet ... all of which work reasonably well – when you DON'T drop it in the toilet at home or at Walmart (sigh). Almost none of the electrical bidets I looked at were built for fat people. So I had to locate a powered bidet which fit on an elongated toilet and could support the weight of a 300-pound person. My BioBidet Bliss BB-2000 has changed my life. I'm easily able to clean myself, even after accidents. Since I'm less stressed about getting to the toilet, I've stopped having accidents! My hemorrhoids have vanished and I'm able to easily handle ALL aspects of toilet hygiene.[1]

Although many types of bidet are a very functional addition to the toilet, it is in some ways more accurate to compare bidets to the shower or tub. Anyone who has mobility problems and finds it difficult to get into a bathtub, or is afraid of slipping in the shower, may find some bidets excellent solutions for crucial parts of their personal hygiene. A bidet offers a new level of comfort and independence for such people, in some instances helping them to avoid some difficult or painful disrobing for bathing.

Bidet toilet seats are a godsend to people with bad backs! I need to get here more often. I was recently affected by my bad back. Degenerative disc disease per 4 docs. I'm 62 years old, I ain't gonna ask my wife to wipe my ass. So I got 1 of those bidet toilet seats. All I can say is thank god and pass the ammunition. Get over the he-man shit...it has nothing to do with that. I now tease the wife and ask her if she's springtime fresh! I tell everyone who visits that it's my second most favorite seat in the house. P.S. It's also heated. [12]

As women age, the lining of the vaginal and bladder skin becomes thin and more easily irritated, requiring more gentle care. This may predispose a woman to bladder and vaginal infections. As men age they are susceptible to similar infections. The bidet is excellent for reducing the likelihood of bacteria being inadvertently introduced into these sensitive areas. [102,191]

Care Givers

Care givers who must keep elderly or handicapped people clean and healthy will find the bidet a godsend. The automatic washing functions of many modern bidets will trivialize what is often considered to be a difficult and unpleasant task. Portable, hand-held devices can give crucial clean ability and flexibility to caregivers in these situations.

The water spray group reported significantly greater convenience and higher overall satisfaction compared with the sitz bath group. At the end of the 4-week postoperative follow-up period, 90% of patients in the watery spray group and 93% of patients in the sitz bath group showed complete wound healing. There were no significant differences in postoperative complications between groups. Conclusion: Our results demonstrate that the water spray method could provide a safe and reliable alternative to the sitz bath for post-hemorrhoidectomy care. Furthermore, the water spray method could be used instead of the sitz bath as a more convenient and satisfactory form of treatment. [42]

In addition to the impact of urinary incontinence on the individual, the condition is assumed to create "spillover" effects among family, other caregivers, and society at large. Noelker found the presence of urinary incontinence to be associated with stress in the primary caregiver as evidenced by perceived care and economic burdens; doubts about care giving; feelings of guilt or anger; reports of health deterioration of the caregiver; and negative effects on family relationships and other social activities. Urinary incontinence is seen as one of several factors contributing to caregiver "breaking point" and the related decision to seek nursing home care. [175]

To shorten the time for a home care worker to help with hygiene, the toilet seat bidet is a good solution and possibly appreciated by the care recipient as well. [256]

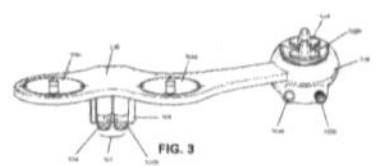

Care of The Genitalia

Both men and women can have a problem cleaning off after peeing. In the best of times there are always a few drops of urine that must be absorbed by the clothing. It is why I wear underpants - to avoid irrevocably staining my trousers. "No matter how much you jiggle and squeeze, those last few drops always go down your knees!" This is an age-old problem for men. Some bidets have an extra spray that is designed to wash the genitals from front to back, and certainly all the handheld units have flexibility to wash off any residual urine.

Live like a king with this dick bidet! Wash and dry your undercarriage with every trip to the toilet. Men, ask yourselves, "is my cock really as clean as it could be?" I mean, you wash your hands after using public restrooms (or at least you should, you filthy bastards) so why wouldn't you give your Rob Thomas a quick cleaning while you're at it? With this new high-tech urinal you'll be able to do just that.[21]

Cleansing with fresh running water daily by using a bidet is a more effective and less irritating way to achieve the highest level of personal hygiene.[37] The bidet also provides very effective feminine hygiene during menstrual periods, and may give women a greater sense of freshness and confidence. Most physicians agree that products such as douches, feminine hygiene deodorants and moist cloth towelettes may cause harm; by irritating the delicate tissues of the urinary meatus and vaginal opening, and by harming beneficial bacteria which inhabit the vaginal environment, thus predisposing woman to infection.[276]

We conducted our original self-completed questionnaire survey on a total of 305 women who came to our urology department as an outpatient from March 2014 to September 2014. They were asked to fill in the questionnaire on their experience of usage as well as how and where they were using the washing function of the toilet seat. The effective response rate was 95.4%. Seventy-nine (230) individuals were using the warm-water washing toilet seat. There was no significant difference in age between the usage group and the non-use group. The purposes of use after defection, for defecation induction, and after urination were 90.4, 41.3, and 40.4%, respectively. Regarding the kinds of washing, a strong tendency for the use of the anal washing function to induce defection and after defecation was observed, whereas a tendency was observed for the use of the bidet function after urination and for washing the vagina... many individuals were using the washing function for the purpose of inducing defection and after urination.[194]

The vagina, located close to the anus. It can easily get soiled when stool and mucus of the large intestine adhere around your anus after doing your business. You can wash away stool and mucus of the large intestine by washing your anus and nearby area with a spray seat after doing your business. On the other hand, you can not solve your problems just by washing your private parts with a bidet, for harmful bacteria are also growing in your vagina, especially when your private parts get stuffy and less clean as a result of wearing restrictive clothing. By the way, even those who have balanced vaginal bacteria need some time before their naturally occurring bacteria restore their original balance after washing the inside of their vagina.[193]

Some Western countries have long had a habit of washing the inside of the vagina and this habit is criticized due to the fact that "vaginal douching" affects the balance of healthy bacteria in the vagina. When you suffer from itching in your private parts, you should reduce friction caused by your clothes or panty liner. You can also make use of a bidet, but when you use the bidet function, you should wash with soft streams for a short period. Washing thoroughly with strong streams will not stop your itching in the long run.[193]

The Water Jet Controversy

Repeated hitting of the anus by water stream could potentially cause injury to the anal canal epithelium and lead to development of fissure-in-ano. As the water stream is emanating from the backside of the toilet commode, the possible injury, if any, would be on the anterior anal canal.   Results: In this study, 165 patients were prospectively enrolled. Male/female ratio was 96/69, and the mean age was 36.3 11.2 years. The anterior fissure-in-ano in the study group was 55.9% (47/84), while it was 17.3 % (14/81) in the control group (P < 0.0001, odds ratio: 6.08, 95% CI: 2.96 - 12.47].   Conclusions: Water used as a single sharp stream to cleanse after defecation in toilet commodes is hazardous and should be avoided.[47]

Users with genital or anal discomfort prefer to use a bidet and there is a correlation with subjects having urological infections, vulvar pruritus and also hemorrhoids. A warm water jet of low or medium pressure was able to reduce anal resting pressure up to 14 mmHg.[49]

The studies above also suggest that the strength of the water flow of the bidets used might be part of the problem. A sharp strong single water jet is not advised for ailing flesh. I personally use a handheld bidet (vegetable sprayer) that has about 30 small jets running at 10-35 PSI, much lower than most urban water pressures. Placed tightly against my anus it greatly induces defecation as suggested in the first study above. Before and after defecation it cleans my anal area quite well spraying slightly farther away and at very low pressure.

I get quick and easy washing of my whole anal area as needed using multiple small jets, each one relatively weak in water pressure. I spray my handheld bidet from the front because I had sanitary problems otherwise. My ability to spray at an angle of my choosing is incredibly helpful (carelessly used it can also lead to messy smelly disasters). For 16 years I have had no problems at all. For details about my process see the **Appendix**.

As a child my family and I would always go on a caravan holiday to the south of France once a year. One particular time, while driving through France, my family stopped at a very small hotel overnight. This hotel had a bidet and when I asked my father naively what the toilet looking sink thing was for he explained it was "for washing your family jewels". Flash forward 10 or so years to a teenage me explaining to someone at a party that "in France they have a special sink just for washing your jewelry." My family has yet to let me live it down.[23]

Various other studies in this book have also commented on the dangers of wash water spraying fecal contamination on the genitalia. It is important that bidets have the option to wash from the front to the back (or vertically) which can eliminate fecal matter contaminating the genetalia. For details about my eliminative process see the **Appendix**.

Water is the best and healthiest way to clean just about everything, says Donnica Moore, MD, host of the podcast In The Ladies Room, and women's health expert in Chester, NJ. If you think about it, when we use dry toilet paper to clean our most sensitive and almost dirtiest areas of our body, that doesn't really make a lot of sense. Our hands are the germiest parts of our bodies, but bidets can be used hands free. So, you may spread fewer germs cleaning yourself with a bidet after going to the bathroom.[50]

According to Dr. Moore, bidets could come in handy during a woman's period, when one may "feel like a mess down there." (Obviously the vagina is self-cleaning, but period blood can get messy.) Compared to most "feminine wipes," which often contain ingredients that can irritate your vulvar skin, a bidet just contains water. Plus, bidets could also be helpful to clean up after sex, Dr. Moore says. "Especially if you enjoy morning sex, and don't have the time to take a complete shower," she says.[50]

Pregnancy

If you have decreased range of motion or mobility due to pregnancy (or an injury), then reaching behind yourself to wipe can be difficult, Dr. Moore says. "You have this big obstruction that changes your center of gravity and can interfere with being able to reach where you need to reach," she says. Or if you recently gave birth and are in pain, using a bidet could be very practical in that sense. Another thing about wiping: you might have heard that wiping front to back is crucial for preventing a UTI, and the same goes for using a bidet. "Make sure you leave the water in the right direction," Dr. Moore says.[50]

Among 212 subjects, 67 (32.0%) women responded that they used bidet toilet. The incidence of preterm birth before 37 weeks of gestation was significantly higher in the users compared to the non-users (86.8% vs. 72.8%). Interestingly, the rate of late preterm birth (GA 34+0-36+6 weeks) in the users was more than twice than the non-users (43.4% vs. 20.6%).[51]

Of 1,293 women who responded to the questionnaire, 63.3% were users of the bidet toilet. The incidence of preterm birth was 15.8% among bidet users and 16.0% among nonusers (adjusted OR 1.04, 95% confidence interval [CI] 0.72-1.48). Additionally, no association was found between bidet toilet use and bacterial vaginosis (adjusted OR 0.96, 95% CI 0.70-1.33). CONCLUSION: Normal use of the bidet toilet by pregnant women poses no clinical health risk for preterm birth and bacterial vaginosis.[52]

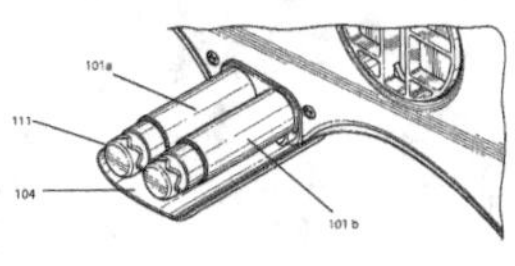

FIG. 5

Lavage using electric warm-water toilet seat units has gained wide use as an appliance for maintaining cleanliness of the perianal region after defecation, and for prevention or improvement of constipation and hemorrhoids by stimulating the rectal region with warm water to promote your anodermal blood circulation. As pregnancy progresses flexibility and mobility decrease, and in the last few months you may find that bending and reaching for normal bathroom related activities is greatly decreased. A bidet can eliminate the need for you to reach behind you or bend forward repeatedly in order to clean yourself after a bowel movement.[87]

According to Ob-gyn Michele M. Hakakha, MD "Hemorrhoids are a sure bet when a woman becomes pregnant. They often occur with constipation and the straining that ensues in an attempt to have a bowel movement. And we all know that constipation is one of the most common complaints in pregnancy".[87]

Very few women make it through pregnancy without developing hemorrhoids, and these can be very painful at times. The pressure of the growing baby can lead to pressure in the lower pelvic area that can contribute to hemorrhoids. Bowel movements may become more difficult as pregnancy progresses and the fetus presses on the bowels. The straining required during natural childbirth can also cause hemorrhoids to develop. A bidet can be invaluable for any woman who has developed hemorrhoids.[87]

A pregnant woman undergoes many physical changes, as well as changes in her body chemistry, that may make it more difficult to keep her genital area clean and odor-free. It also helps to cleanse harmful bacteria that may cause vaginal and bladder infections, thus minimizing the need for medications that could endanger her baby.[279-80] **Normal use of the bidet toilet by pregnant women poses no clinical health risk for preterm birth and bacterial vaginosis.**[42]

A bidet can be very available and quick to use for pregnant women, especially late in their pregnancy when mobility may be decreased. Pre-delivery patients were advised to use the bidet each time they used the toilet, and the importance of drying the perineum was stressed (many bidets can air dry).[43]

After giving birth, many women return home with vaginal tears or surgical incisions such as episiotomies that need hygiene and care to avoid infection. Bidets are an excellent aid for genital TLC during the healing process.[132]

Bacterial counts in the stored water in household units of electric warm-water lavage toilet seats were 3-times higher, compared to units in public facilities, suggesting a correlation with the turnover of the water in the tank.[53] If the bidet is used daily this should not be a problem. Most high-end bidets have self-cleaning features for both the spray head and the bowl. When deciding on a unit, this should be a significant consideration.

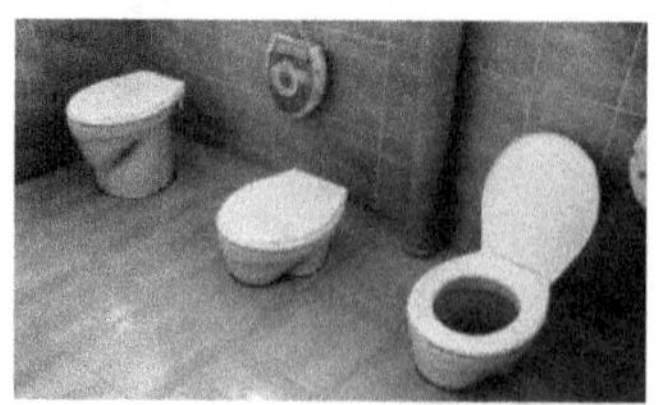

Infant Care/Potty Training

Infants and toddlers need a lot of bottom cleaning, and anything that makes this process faster and easier is generally desirable. Many bidets can be used for washing out cloth diapers and any other changing materials. As your child ages, the bidet can also become an integral part of his or her potty-training, making this difficult part of growing up much easier for everyone involved. My granddaughter Clara's comments on their new bidet at the beginning of this book are quite revealing about how pleasurable a bidet can be for a child.

The benefits can be many: children can avoid constipation as a result of toilet training (see **Health, Constipation**). They need help in keeping themselves clean, and generally are happier when their bowel movements are a pleasant experience. Additionally, a child's tender skin benefits from many of the points made in this section.

It was wonderful to confidently bathe our baby. As for Sabrina... she loved it! The soft spray did not frighten her as the shower did and we didn't have to worry about dropping her. As for diaper changing... what a dream come true. Sabrina was prone to diaper rash unless I washed her bottom at changings. Doing that over the sink meant I got soaked, my arms got tired and it was not at all comfortable for her either. With the ShowerBaby, I can clean her the way nature intended, with clean running water. Susan & Adam K.[10]

Bidets are a good stepping stone for kids. Good personal hygiene is something we all want for our kids. Washing your bottom after every "use" is a good reminder for children to follow when they perform proper bathroom hygiene. It will continuously be used to help them to develop great personal hygiene habits. Personal hygiene is important for children and it will help prevent them from getting sick by eliminating fecal matter and bacteria.[28]

I bathed my baby in one in Italy. There was no tub in the hotel, and she just fit. During a year in Paris, we used ours for washing smalls and feet, as well as the intended parts. Our flat had only one toilet for four people, and I will admit that my husband and son used it as a urinal occasionally. I miss it terribly. Barbara Murray, Brookline, Massachusetts[23]

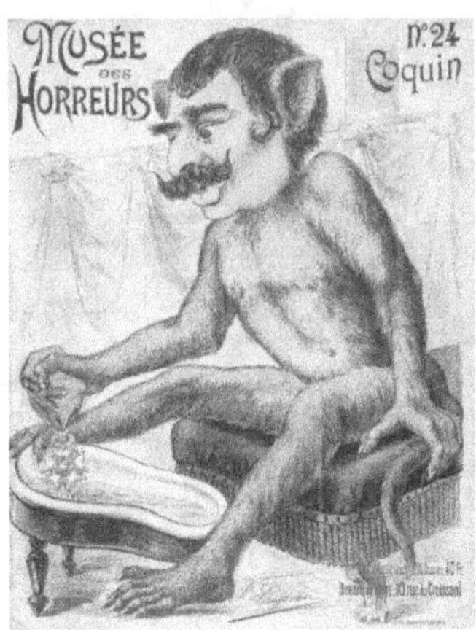

Coquin: Musée des horreurs

Physical Intimacy - Sexual Intercourse

Using fresh running water before and after intercourse can play an important role in keeping you fresh and clean naturally.[50] Proper personal hygiene plays an important role in getting close with your mate. Smell, feel, and cleanliness are all important prerequisites for intimacy. Rinsing with the Bidet both before and after intercourse by both partners can be a wonderful aid to your love life.

Compared to most "feminine wipes," which often contain ingredients that can irritate your vulvar skin, a bidet just contains water. Plus, bidets could also be helpful to clean up after sex, Dr. Moore says. "Especially if you enjoy morning sex, and don't have the time to take a complete shower," she says.[50]

Well between the bidet and the hand held I think I am in love. Again I found that washing and rinsing the anus using the hand held could also be stimulating. Having never realized how stimulated ones anus could become. Who thought a shot of water to your backside could make you aroused? So you can only imagine my surprise and delight when washing and rinsing my female genitalia. Again much like my first bidet experience I got more than I would have ever imagined.[12]

First time I used a bidet was in Jamaica. I sat down, cranked up the fountain spray between my legs to almost my chin, and used the water to brush my teeth! We were newly married and became addicted. Great for pre-love body wash...in all those important crevices and sensitive places where lips and tongues roam. When the house was in party mode, twosomes of gals going for a pee might sorta co-pee, one on the bidet and the other on the toilet, with both using the bidet for that clean and ready security. As a guy, it is a great bag washer, and bum washer. We keep liquid soap on hand, and it is simply nice to always be clean. Bidets keep your undershorts clean, the odors down, and sexuality tweaked and at the ready. If you really want a quickie, the bidet is quicker than the shower.[216]

If your toilet doesn't have a bidet or an inbuilt tap there are other solutions. We live in North America and use soap and watering can(the ones you use to water plants) to clean our genitals. Before sitting on the toilet seat, we fill up the watering can (you can adjust the warmth of the water from the tap) Toilet paper is mostly to use initially before the actual washing and afterwards to wipe dry. I can't imagine myself walking around with ..... in my genitals all day. This is why i carry with me a bottle of water to the public washroom or if i forgot, i soak some toilet paper or towel, maybe also add a little soap on it and wipe with it.[216]

I can't believe in the year 2005 there's still people who don't EVEN KNOW what a bidet is and who are... SCARED of it! I read once that American people think they are the world's cleanest (not to mention, the world's most civilized)... well they're so clean and civilized, that they keep the most delicate parts of their body (not only the anus ok?) dirty!! Wow it's terrible! I don't even want to think about sex among dirty persons like them![12]

Islamic Toilet Etiquette

In relation to the grooming activities following the use of a toilet, Gallagher separates the users in two categories "the wipers and the washers". The Turkish culture belongs mainly to the washers' category. Muslims, Japanese and continental Europeans are all 'washers', mostly using a bidet after passing motion. For the Muslims, this is also a religious requirement, while for the others; washing gives them a greater sense of hygiene. In the Muslim faith, this washing is concerned with cleanliness and purity of body and soul, and can be applied to both sitting and squatting toilet postures. This comes from the fact that the Islamic culture gives an important role to water in praying, to purify the body and the soul.[125]

Islamic toilet etiquette is a set of personal hygiene rules in Islam followed when going to the toilet. The only issue that the Qur'an mentions is the one of washing one's hands (verse 5:6). Issues of chirality (bodily symmetry), such as whether one uses the left or right hand, and which foot is used to step into or out of toilet areas. The anus must be washed with water using the left hand after defecating. Similarly, the penis and vulva must be washed with water with the left hand after urinating. This washing is known as istinja. The Qur'an suggests that one should wash one's hands as well, which is discussed in verse 5:6.[291]

The Khalifah Project notes that Muslims must 'enter the toilet with the left foot and leave with the right foot'. It is considered 'detestable' to stand while urinating. After using the toilet, purification of the peritoneal area by running water ('Istinja') is required. Therefore, to comply with some religious beliefs, bidets or basins should be provided in each toilet to enable people to wash themselves with running water.[126]

In our religion Muslims wash every time when visiting the toilet - both for urination and excretion. We have to be extra particular about keeping the body and clothes free from impurities (urine, stool) otherwise the 5 daily prayers would be invalid. To assist in this, men always urinate sitting down so that urine is not (accidentally) splashed on the seat, floor, clothes and body. As people have said, tissue is not really enough, a combination of tissue and water is the best method. In Muslim nations - hand-held bidets or watering cans are common.[12]

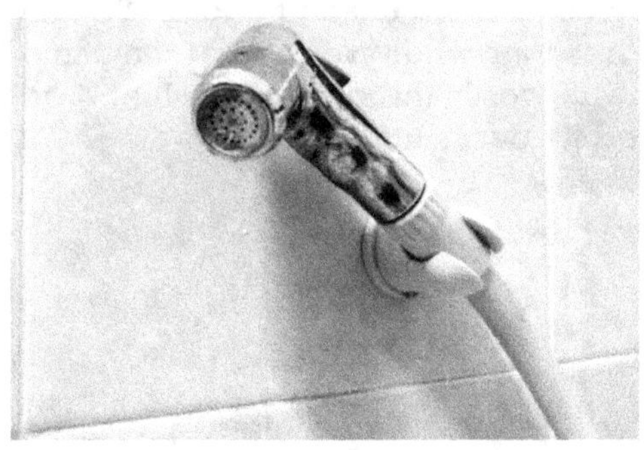

Muslim Shattaf

Bidets Can Eliminate Bad Odors

Ninety-nine percent of the gases that make up your farts don't smell. Farts are mostly oxygen, nitrogen, carbon dioxide, hydrogen and methane. The other one percent stinks—it's made of sulfuric compounds. On average, people fart between thirteen and twenty-one times a day. Basically, if you're not farting all day, there's probably something wrong with you.[297]

SUNDAY POOP

Sunday should be a day of rest,
but often it is when our sphincter is put to its greatest test.
A weekend of eating junk and throwing back some beers,
leaves rancid smelling bathrooms that have put men in tears.
There is nothing to be ashamed of if this applies to you,
so have some pride when the next person
walks in the bathroom and says phew.
For your stink will be lingering for hours,
it will be more eternal than the stonehenge towers.
So after the first round of football games come to a close,
run to that bathroom and enjoy
the sweet smell out your nose! – StinkerThinker[306]

The more advanced TSBs, French bidets, (and Clos O Mat) have gotten pretty effective in eliminating unpleasant smells from the toilet bowl. The same fan that blows you dry after elimination, works in reverse to suck the malodorous air out of the toilet bowl. This fan then directs this foul air into a cartridge of activated charcoal. Oxygen has activated this carbon and caused it to develop millions of pores, which greatly expands the surface area of the charcoal. This process is called adsorption, where that huge carbon surface area attracts the smelly molecules which stick to it. The air that comes through the filtration system is much cleaner and without unwanted odors. This is truly deodorizing the air, rather than simply covering up the odors in your bathroom.[87]

Less toilet paper and cleaner air in the bathroom! We bought the C100 and it's wonderful! It immediately reduced our need for toilet paper and the air deodorizer is very effective at eliminating odors. We only have one bathroom so that's a breath of fresh air when it's used at the same time as the shower. The deodorizer alone is worth the cost of washlet. The heated seat can be nice, though we turned it down a little.[1]

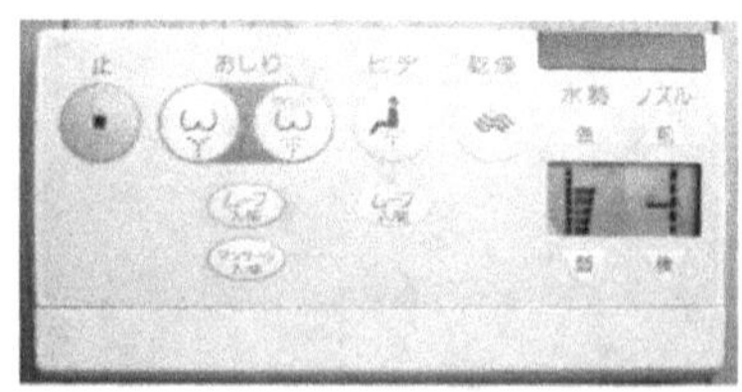

Wireless Bidet Control Panel

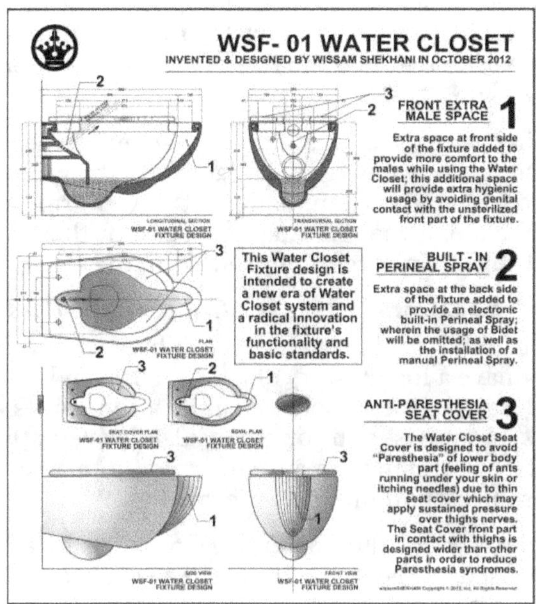

Bidet Health

Medically, the bidet offers notable benefits as a result of increased cleanliness, the therapeutic effect of water on damaged or irritated skin, and increased circulation brought about by the massaging effect of a pressurized stream of water. The following material usually applies to all bidets.

[Hans Maurer, inventor of the Clos O Mat,1983] The most effective factor in promoting sales was quite unmistakably the word-of-mouth propaganda coming from satisfied customers. One could rely on this oral publicity right from the very first customer onwards - because everyone making use of a Clos-O-Mat very rapidly became a champion of this form of intimate hygiene. Among the customers who were the most enthusiastic advocates of the device were those who thanks to the Clos-O-Mat were able to get some relief from, and alleviation of, such ailments as hemorrhoids.[24]

In countries like Japan and Korea, where almost every home has an electronic bidet-toilet, it is expected that the move to a diagnostic toilet would be a logical step... At the Wonju campus of Yonsei University in Korea a toilet has been developed that will undertake pathology tests on wastes. The toilet is also the site for a tele-health consultation where vital signs can be taken. When a person steps up to the toilet their weight is recorded. The toilet is equipped with devices for blood pressure, oximetry and other measures.[68]

A low total viable count of bacterial P. aeruginosa TVC (≤ 1/mL) in the spray waters from both on-demand and tank-type warm-water bidet toilet seats

showed low bacterial contamination, although there was an increase in....
growth of biofilms, inside in the warm-water bidet toilet seats.... Collectively
our findings demonstrate that hygienic safety of warm-water bidet toilet seats
is being maintained overall.[120]

The health-preserving benefits of bidets are dependent on the quality of the water
used. Bidets with separate water supplies (generally high-end TSBs) can be an
additional source of bacterial contamination. If their warm water reservoirs are
not used frequently enough the chlorine antiseptic in the water can eventually
evaporate. Some advanced units routinely self-clean the water supply.

Traditional Bidets and Sitz Baths

The many medical benefits of classic and French bidets are very straightforward.
These types of bidet have a long history of medical use, and bidets are considered
as Durable Medical Equipment by some insurance companies due to their many
therapeutic benefits. (I suppose you could consider a constantly soiled derriere as
an illness or injury.) Searching for any information on the bidet on our FDA
website, I found absolutely nothing. Zero information.

Definition: "Durable Medical Equipment" Durable medical equipment is any
medical equipment used in the home to aid in a better quality of living. It is a
benefit included in most insurances.[275]

The classic bidet (and French bidets that can be stopped up) can be used as sitz
baths. A sitz bath (also called a hip bath) is a type of bath in which only the hips
and buttocks are soaked in water or saline solution. Its name comes from the
German verb sitzen, meaning to sit. These bidets are actually better then the
standard sitz bath, because they can control the temperature of the water as well
as constantly replacing the water for better hygiene. Some models also have a
water jet for improved water circulation.

A sitz bath is recommended for patients who have had surgery in the area of the
rectum or genitals. It eases painful genitals, the pain of hemorrhoids and prostate
infections, as well as uterine cramps. It also helps to minimize the discomfort
caused by infections of the prostate, vagina, or bladder. Sitz baths are also used to
treat inflammatory bowel diseases.[42,131-2]

A bidet has been proposed as a replacement for the sitz bath. Like a sitz bath,
it brings water into contact with the perineum. However, the high force of
water from commercially used electronic bidets may harm the anus. We
developed a new electronic bidet and evaluated its effects on anal resting
pressure compared with a warm sitz bath... The maximal increase and
minimal decrease were not significantly different. The rectal temperature was
not elevated, and the water temperature decreased significantly with the sitz
bath ($p < 0.001$). Conclusions -- Our new electronic bidet may reduce the anal
resting pressure much like a warm sitz bath does.[133]

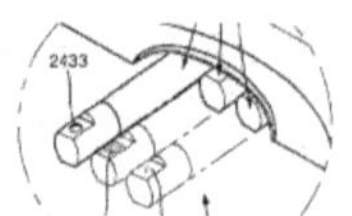

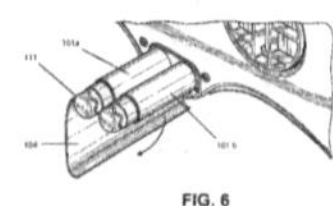

Disease Prevention

A meta-analysis in hygiene based on observed and self-reported information found that rarely more than 50% of the people wash their hands after the use of a toilet. A UK-wide study of hygiene published by the BBC found that 32% of British men washed their hands and 64% of the women. Estimates based on a meta-analysis concluded that improved hygiene could reduce the rate of gastrointestinal illness by 31% and respiratory illness by 21%. This suggests that a more hygienic alternative for toilet paper may also potentially improve overall health, using a bidet for example, removes the part of the toileting sequence where the user has almost direct physical contact between his/her hands and the feces he/she tries to remove. Most people value their health and the environment and yet persist in behaving in ways that undermine it.[66]

Almost 80 percent of all infectious diseases are passed on by human contact and only about half of us actually wash our hands after using the bathroom—making hands-free bidets a safer alternative all around. "If you don't have to use your hands at all then there is less chance of passing or coming in contact with a virus".[20]

The benefits of cleanliness discussed in the last section can have direct benefits on maintaining health and preventing disease. There are other less direct health benefits of bidets.

My wife has very bad cases both of Crohn's disease and colitis. Had I known that converting our existing toilet to a bidet would be so ridiculously simple and inexpensive, I would have done it over a decade ago! I wish I had known about USABIDET products. My wife now enjoys her new Peri-Jett device. The pH balancing effects in the OTC Peri-Jett solution have alleviated a lot of the pain she endured up to 25 times/day for almost 15 years. She appreciates the deodorizing effect of the Peri-Jett the most. Christian S. Canton, GA.[41]

[USABidet vendor's comment] The Perijett has also proved to be an essential hygienic fixture for (i) those with a limited range of motion due to arm, hip, or back surgery - especially rotator cuff surgery, (ii) elderly and bariatric patients, (iii) anyone needing a raised toilet seat, (iv) incontinence. We recently received a GSA contract award (#36F79718D0483) to provide Perijett hygiene assist devices to VA.[41]

A scientific study found that the frequency of bathing (at least 5 times or more weekly) is more important than the mode of bathing (tub vs. shower) in effectively treating dry skin.[192] Similarly, the frequent use of a bidet may greatly reduce dry skin around the anus, and would potentially also prevent dry skin around the penis. I personally have not had any skin problems in my perianal area, whereas the rest of my skin does continue to have its problems. Water, absorbed through bathing, will hydrate skin but will rapidly be lost to evaporation unless a topical occlusive agent is applied to prevent moisture loss through the skin.[192]

Bathe to relieve dry skin. Some simple changes to your bath time can reduce (or alleviate) dry, itchy skin and prevent dry, itchy from becoming a serious problem. Here's what you can do: Stop using bar soap. Replace it with a gentle, creamy, fragrance-free cleanser or emollient. Use warm (not hot) water. Hot water strips skin of its natural oils, which can increase skin dryness. Use a soft cloth to wash your skin. A buff puff or bath brush can irritate your skin. Keep your bath or shower short. You may find that you don't need to bathe every day. When you bathe, keep it short. Take a 10-minute bath or shower. Pat water gently from your skin after bathing, but leave a bit of water on your skin. Having some water on your skin when you apply moisturizer (next step) helps hydrate your skin. Apply a creamy, fragrance-free moisturizer formulated for dry skin within 3 minutes of bathing and throughout the day. This helps ease the dryness and restore your skin's protective barrier.[191]

Skin Infection

We do know that to prevent perineal skin injury, it is helpful to prevent excessive skin hydration, minimize the interaction of urine and feces, minimize local microorganisms, and maintain skin near its physiologic pH.[135]

(Japan) There is a relation between childhood leukemia and the use of electric appliances... Statistically significant risk ratios (OR) were the following: the highest category of hair drier use by mother during conception with OR of 1.86; the longest TV watching by mother with OR of 1.73; the low category of electric toilet shower by mother with OR of 0.46; the longest TV watching by child with OR of 2.40; the low hair drier category with OR 0.43... The low category of the use of toilet shower, like an electric bidet, showed a significantly lower risk against the lowest category including no use.[134]

This suggests that using an electric bidet halves the risk of childhood leukemia in Japan. Additionally, consider the potential effects of medications used for the sore or chafed anus and genital area. Remember that all medications affect our bodies and may interact with other medications we may be taking. It is always best to minimize our use of medications by acting to maintain genital and perianal health, and the bidet can help achieve this goal.

As we age, our skin requires more tender care, and a bidet is an ideal solution. Where the bidet really shines is in spot cleaning, washing as needed, and requires no soap. Tap water coming through the bidet helps keep skin irritations to a minimum, and infections clean and relatively germ free.[37,92-97] Gentle air drying without paper or rubbing greatly aids this.

Aging skin experiences increased dryness (allowing cracks in which bacteria colonize) and slower recovery from the effects of alkaline substances... Skin should be cleansed gently without high alkalinity (as in some bar soaps) or rubbing (which denudes fragile skin), patted or air dried, moisturized after bathing, and protected with a barrier.[143]

Perineal-rectal care is defined as skin care to the region between the vulva and anus in the female and scrotum and anus in the male. Perineal-rectal care is essential to prevent infection and promote comfort but is complicated by the anatomical location. In addition, no standardized perineal-rectal care approach exists.[136]

A common theme throughout this book is our ignorance of everything related to the health of our "privates." This also applies in many ways to doctors and medicine as well. There are conditions in this area of your body that medicine hasn't significantly addressed and is still struggling to treat effectively. Many general practice doctors avoid this area, or relegate it to the care of nurses. The bidet benefits your genital/perianal health and cleanliness in a more direct effective manner, thus ultimately furthering disease prevention.[76-81]

"Bidets have health benefits?" (Uttered by a proctologist when I told him about this book).[44]

Pruritus Ani
Intense chronic itching in the anal area

Pruritus ani is a common and socially embarrassing condition which is often poorly managed. It is often classified as idiopathic where the symptoms are usually transitory or secondary when a more persistent itch is experienced... the majority of patients presenting with pruritus ani have a dermatosis as the underlying cause of their symptoms and that many of them have developed contact sensitivities to the various topical medications used.[137]

The use of soap, particularly scented ones, should be avoided—warm water alone can be used, and the area should not be scrubbed vigorously during bathing or after toileting. The use of prepared wipes and witch hazel pads should be avoided—unscented toilet paper moistened with warm water is preferable. The region should be patted dry, or a hair dryer on a cool setting should be used.

Although bidets are not commonly used in the United States, commercially available toilet seat covers with bidet functions popularized in Japan have been making inroads into this country, and may provide a less abrasive means of cleansing the perianal region.[129]

The essentials of the treatment of pruritus ani consist of keeping the perianal skin scrupulously clean and dry, while avoiding irritation from over-cleaning. The most important damaging factors are fecal residue, moisture, scratching, steroids, and local anesthetics.[138-40] Bidets can keep the skin clean of fecal residue without soap or medications (see above) and can allow for full drying with air dry features. I personally have found my bidet excellent for quickly eliminating skin irritations and itchiness, even though mine does not have air drying. I use a dedicated wash cloth.

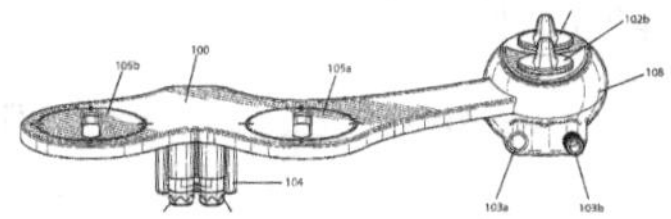

Half of the sufferers in another study had poor or incomplete elimination resulting in frequent soiling and residue. It is important to note that either poor hygiene or overly enthusiastic hygiene can cause Pruritus Ani. Patients tend to worsen the problem by application of many medications and overzealous cleaning with excessive rubbing and use of harsh soaps.[137-39]

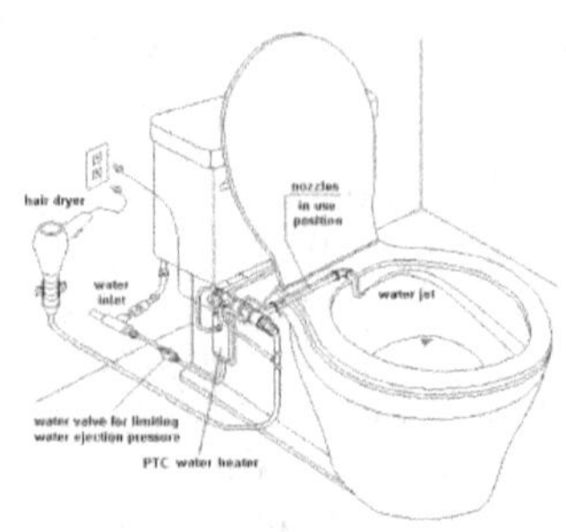

Anal Fissure

painful tears or ulcers in the lining of the anus

An anal fissure is a break or tear in the skin of the anal canal. Anal fissures may be noticed by bright red anal bleeding on toilet paper and undergarments, or sometimes in the toilet. If acute they are painful after defecation. Most anal fissures are caused by stretching of the anal mucosa beyond its capability. Superficial or shallow anal fissures look much like a paper cut, and may be hard to detect upon visual inspection, they will generally self-heal within a couple of weeks.[2]

However, some anal fissures become chronic and deep and will not heal. The result is a non-healing ulcer, which may become infected by fecal bacteria. In adults, fissures may be caused by constipation, the passing of large, hard stools, or by prolonged diarrhea. In older adults, anal fissures may be caused by decreased blood flow to the area. For adults, the following may help prevent anal fissures: Avoiding straining when defecating, Careful anal hygiene after defecation, including using soft toilet paper and/or cleaning with water, if needed the use of sanitary wipes.[2]

Results: Bowel movement was successfully induced in 15 of the 20 patients (75%). Success was not related significantly to injury level, ASIA impairment scale, or ability to voluntarily squeeze. Compared with their usual manner of bowel management, for which they spent more than 30 minutes, time needed for successful bowel movement was shortened in 11 of 13 patients. No complications were observed.[148]

Several studies have established that a single sharp stream of water from a bidet can damage the perianal area. This can easily be avoided. Users these days have complete control over the shape of the stream of water, from single stream to essentially a shower head, as well as how much water flow and temperature. That is why a book like this is necessary, a book that is completely independent and deeply delves into everything bidet.[131]

The anterior fissure-in-ano in the study group was 55.9% (47/84), while it was 17.3 % (14/81) in the control group (P < 0.0001]. Conclusions: Water used as a single sharp stream to cleanse after defecation in toilet commodes is hazardous and should be avoided.[47]

My home water pressure (10-40 psi) is always much weaker than municipal water supplies (often 80-100+ psi). It would be easy to add a water pressure lowering valve, or if you have a bidet with a separate water on/off valve, simply do not fully open it and this will effectively reduce the water pressure. A water pressure of only 10 psi. in my opinion is sufficient to clean, and even initiate defecation.

Dermatitis

Dermatitis is an inflammation of the skin.

The word "dermatitis" is used to describe a number of different skin rashes that are caused by infections, allergies, and irritating substances and range from mild to severe. There are two common forms: Atrophic dermatitis is inherited and usually occurs first when children are infants. Contact dermatitis occurs when the skin comes in contact with something that causes an allergic reaction (allergic contact dermatitis) or injures the skin (irritant contact dermatitis).[127]

A major study found almost no research on what makes perineal skin injuries worse in adults, but did find extensive research on babies' skin problems that may be applied to adults. By removing extrinsic substances from the skin, bidets should help the skin to achieve its physiologic pH. Bidets that offer automatic air-drying prevent excessive skin hydration.

The six extrinsic environmental factors that have been identified and extensively studied in diaper dermatitis are skin wetness, urine, ammonia, feces, local skin pH and microorganisms. Although the complex interactions of the six factors are still not totally defined, we do know that to prevent perineal skin injury, it is helpful to prevent excessive skin hydration, minimize the interaction of urine and feces, minimize local microorganisms, and maintain skin near its physiologic pH. In general, the six extrinsic factors can be extrapolated and applied to the skin care of adults.[135]

The most important form of non-medical management of anal eczema is to improve hygiene to ensure that the perianal area is cleansed of fecal deposits or urine, that irritate the skin, in a way that does not further irritate the skin (e.g. by excessive rubbing or exposure to harsh soaps and detergents or allergens). Instead, bidets (or baths), soft wet washcloths (or cotton balls) or unscented baby wipes are recommended followed by gentle dabbing to dry the area using cotton balls, unbleached, unscented tissue or a soft cloth.[237]

[*Baby-wipe dermatitis: preservative-induced hand eczema in parents and persons using moist towelettes*] RESULTS: A total of 6 women and 3 men with hand eczema were found to be allergic to preservatives found in different brands of moist towelettes used in diaper hygiene. Many were allergic to fragrance materials as well. The eruptions were mostly worse on the thumb and 2 adjacent fingers, with which the item was held. Five of the 9 were parents of infants, although no infant had a problem. Only 1 patient suspected the source.[88]

Dermatitis is a common problem for incontinent patients; a cycle of moisture, friction, bacteria and breakdown can be established. To break this cycle, the clinician must understand the etiology of incontinence dermatitis and choose appropriate skin care products. Healthy skin has a mean acid mantle of 5.5

pH. This natural acidity discourages bacterial colonization and provides a moisture barrier. Aging skin experiences increased dryness (allowing cracks in which bacteria colonizes) and slower recovery from the effects of alkaline substances. Incontinence results in elevated friction coefficient, exposure to moisture, bacteria and ammonia leading to alkaline conditions, and increased enzymatic activity. Skin should be cleansed gently without high alkalinity (as in some bar soaps) or rubbing (which denudes fragile skin), patted or air dried, moisturized after bathing, and protected with a barrier.[143]

It is interesting that this study doesn't even mention the bidet, which is the epitome of gentle, pH-balanced cleansing. Many modern bidets clean the skin without soap or rubbing and have an integral air-dry feature. Of all washing agents, water has the least effect on skin pH, and has similar effects on other indices of skin health.[37] Once renewed, the skin naturally provides its own moisture barrier.

Infections Of The Genitals

Vaginal infection

Vaginitis, also called vulvovaginitis, is an inflammation or infection of the vagina. It can also affect the vulva, which is the external part of a woman's genitals. Vaginitis can cause itching, pain, discharge, and odor. Vaginitis is common, especially in women in their reproductive years. It usually happens when there is a change in the balance of bacteria or yeast that are normally found in your vagina. There are different types of vaginitis, and they have different causes, symptoms, and treatments... You can have vaginitis if you are allergic or sensitive to certain products that you use. Examples include vaginal sprays, douches, spermicides, soaps, detergents, or fabric softeners. They can cause burning, itching, and discharge. If your vaginitis is due to an allergy or sensitivity to a product, you need to figure out which product is causing the problem. [198]

Self-care for Vaginitis:

- Keep your genital area clean and dry when you have vaginitis.
- Avoid soap and just rinse with water to clean yourself.
- Soak in a warm bath -- not a hot one. Dry thoroughly afterward. Pat the area dry, don't rub.
- Avoid using hygiene sprays, fragrances, or powders in the genital area.
Girls and women should also:
- Know how to properly clean their genital area while bathing or showering
- Wipe properly after using the toilet -- always from front to back
  (or use a bidet to properly, completely clean front to back)
Wash thoroughly before and after using the bathroom.[198]

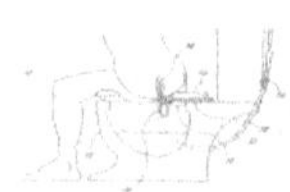

Bidets accomplish everything listed above. Good hygiene is important to prevent this condition. Because vaginal sprays or heavily perfumed soaps can cause vaginal irritation, most doctors advise against these products. The bidet can soothe vaginitis or balanitis symptoms and may help prevent the development of infection by washing the source of the infection away from the genitals. A bidet's ability to thoroughly cleanse with just water makes it a valuable deterrent to irritation, and may thus reduce risks of genital infection. Regular use of the bidet can replace the worry and suffering of infection with soothing comfort and peace of mind.[37,43]

(2017) These findings suggest that positive relations between habitual bidet toilet use and hemorrhoids and urogenital symptoms, except bacterial vaginitis, were due to reverse causation. The incidence of bacterial vaginitis might be caused by bidet toilet use, but the incidence rates were too small to make a definite conclusion, and further studies are needed.[204]   (2018) Cumulative incidence of hemorrhoids and urogenital infections was not significantly increased by habitual use of a bidet toilet.[205]

There have been problems with a few women whose urethra is more proximal to the anus and shorter than that of males. They apparently did not use a strong enough stream of water to properly cleanse (and perhaps did not use the front to back spray on most bidets).

All these 5 women, suspecting its disease connection or according to the advice of a physician, refrained from using the washing system and have since remained symptom-free for months to years. The present observation suggests that Japan's high-tech toilets are not without pitfalls for females whose urethra is more proximal to the anus and shorter than that of males. While cleansing the anus, some water spills over the perineum and vulva, and may presumably contaminate the urethra with enteric bacilli. A strong stream of water for bidet would facilitate the ascent of organisms from the introitus into the bladder. Thus, we have come to suspect that some female users of this "sophisticated" toilet, but not male users, are at risk of developing urinary tract infection.[203]

(2013) RESULTS: Of 1,293 women who responded to the questionnaire, 63.3% were users of the bidet toilet. The incidence of preterm birth was 15.8% among bidet users and 16.0% among nonusers (adjusted OR 1.04, 95% confidence interval [CI] 0.72–1.48). Additionally, no association was found between bidet toilet use and bacterial vaginosis (adjusted OR 0.96, 95% CI 0.70–1.33). **Normal use of the bidet toilet by pregnant women poses no clinical health risk for preterm birth and bacterial vaginosis.**[52]

TSBs, Infection, and Probiotics

There is a controversy in Japan where most people own warm-water cleaning toilets. Early studies found that that some female habitual users of these toilets had less probiotics in their vagina, and this was aggravated by bidet use, which for some can make for poor health of your vagina. Better safe than sorry; it is simple and easy health insurance for female users of warm-water cleaning toilets to periodically take a probiotic supplement.

Aim: Warm-water cleaning toilets, or 'bidet toilets', are one of the most popular household goods in Japan. However, a recent large-scale survey raised questions about the relationship between bidet toilet use and bacterial vaginitis as reflecting bacterial vaginosis with inflammation... Normal microflora (Lactobacillus species) was not present in 42.86% of bidet toilet users, compared to 8.77% of non-users. Fecal bacteria were detected in 50 of the 268 cases (18.66%), 46 cases in users (92%) and only 4 cases in non-users (8%). Contamination by other pathogens was 4 to 6 times higher in users than in non-users... Conclusion: Habitual use of bidet toilets aggravates vaginal microflora, either by depriving normal microflora or facilitating opportunistic infection of fecal bacteria and other microorganisms.[199] [2010]

(2016) Bacterial vaginosis is said to be the most common vaginal syndrome affecting fertile, premenopausal, and pregnant women. Bacterial vaginosis is associated with important adverse health conditions and infectious complications. Therapy with oral or local recommended antibiotics is often associated with failure and high rates of recurrences. The dominance of lactobacilli in healthy vaginal microbiota and its depletion in bacterial vaginosis has given rise to the concept of oral or vaginal use of probiotic Lactobacillus strains for the treatment and prevention of bacterial vaginosis.[200]

Conclusions - Vaginally administered or orally ingested Lactobacillus is able to colonize the vaginal ecosystem. Controlled intervention studies regarding the effect of such colonization on vulvovaginal candidiasis are promising but few... In the meantime, health care providers should discuss potential benefits with affected patients while clarifying the current lack of conclusive evidence.[201]

The predominant growth of Gram-negative germs and the presence of Candida albicans on the external genitalia was significantly higher in women who never used the bidet. No significant differences was however observed in the prevalence of single bacterial species between the two groups of women. Conclusion: Our data suggest that the methods of genital ablution can influence the bacterial flora residing between the genitocrural folds. **The use of the bidet could have a protective effect** against infection of the external mucosa and may reduce the incidence of episodes of infective vulvo-vaginitis which are a common problem in sexually active women.[219]

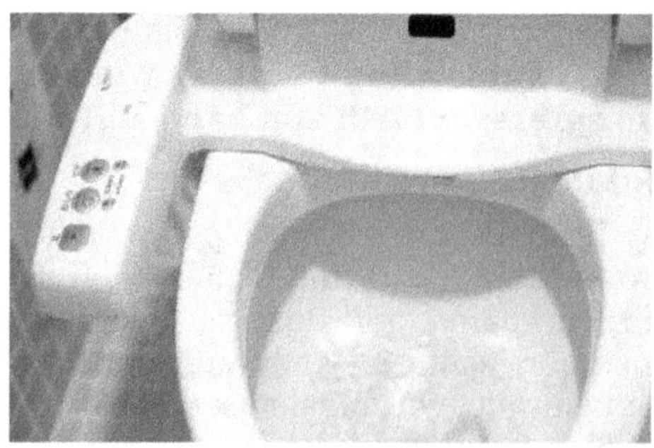

The nozzle emerges from the middle overhang when in use

Men's Balanitis

Males can get an inflammation of the foreskin and/or head of the penis called balanitis, which usually occurs in uncircumcised men and is caused by poor hygiene. It is a common condition, affecting approximately 1 in every 25 boys and 1 in 30 uncircumcised males at some time in their life. This inflammation can be caused by a bacterial, fungal, or viral infection, caustic soaps, or failure to properly rinse soap off while bathing. Balanitis can be uncomfortable and sometimes painful, but it is not usually serious. An antifungal or antibiotic medication may be prescribed. Major causes are infection (either bacterial or fungal), harsh soaps, or not rinsing soap off properly while bathing.[194]

Good hygiene is important to prevent this condition. Because harsh or heavily perfumed soaps can cause irritation, most doctors advise against these products. The bidet can soothe balanitis symptoms and may help prevent the development of infection by keeping the source of the infection away from the genitals. A bidet's ability to thoroughly cleanse with just water makes it a valuable deterrent to irritation, and may thus reduce risks of genital infection. Regular use of the bidet can replace the worry and suffering of infection with soothing comfort and peace of mind.

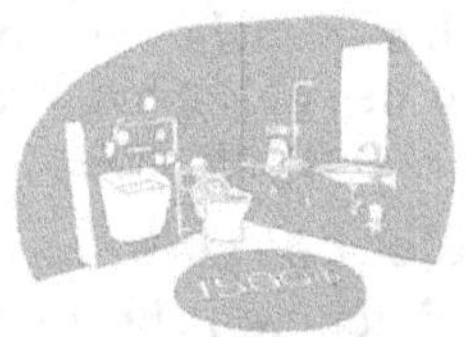

Urinary Tract Infections

I'm sorry, but everyone who is saying using a bidet will give you a UTI is in error. I am an American woman living in Japan, where bidets are the norm, and I have never in 6+ years had a UTI from using a bidet, though I used to get them constantly before coming over here. The water the bidet uses is clean, as another poster mentioned, and while it's aimed forward, it also is not aimed directly into the urethra, and washes the general area. The ones here can spray in either a straight stream or can move side to side. There are also 2 angles you can choose from, for #1 or #2. You can adjust the water pressure so that it isn't very strong. I have saved a lot of TP, and my lady parts have never felt cleaner or smelled better. At first, I laughed at these silly toilets. Now, I am apparently a bidet ambassador. I'm sure European bidet users will confirm that they don't get UTIs this way either... When I wipe after bidet-ing (ha, I invented a new verb), there is rarely anything but water on the paper, usually one wipe with far less paper is necessary. When I visit my family in the US, I can say I definitely feel grosser using just TP alone.[84]

Female, here! My bidet has the same nozzle as a kitchen sink sprayer. So, I can move it to the front or backside. I use a towel to dry off. The only time I use toilet paper is when I am not at home. Not sure why it's not a common thing in the US. Someone said something about UTI's. I began using a bidet because I would get them frequently. I haven't had one in the two years I have used it.[84]

Urinary tract infections typically occur when bacteria enter the urinary tract through the urethra and begin to multiply in the bladder. Although the urinary system is designed to keep out such microscopic invaders, these defenses sometimes fail. When that happens, bacteria may take hold and grow into a full-blown infection in the urinary tract. Each type of UTI may result in more-specific signs and symptoms, depending on which part of your urinary tract is infected.[193]

Kidney infection (acute pyelonephritis)   Upper back and side (flank) pain, High fever, Shaking and chills, Nausea, Vomiting
Bladder (Interstitial cystitis)   Pelvic pressure; Lower abdomen discomfort; Frequent, painful urination; Blood in urine
Urethra (urethritis) Burning with urination, Discharge.[193]

Steps to reduce the risk of urinary tract infections (especially in women) include washing the skin around the vagina (genitals) and anus daily, taking showers rather than tub baths, and wiping from front to back after a bowel movement to prevent bacteria in the anal region from spreading to the vagina and urethra. Most TSB bidets can wash from front to back without any need of wiping. Empty your bladder soon after intercourse. Also, drink a full glass of water to help flush bacteria. Avoid potentially irritating feminine products. Using deodorant sprays or other feminine products, such as douches and powders, in the genital area can irritate the urethra.[193,276] Regular use of the bidet to keep things clean is essential. Water alone is often sufficient to keep things clean.[93-5]

Kidney infection (acute pyelonephritis)

Kidney infection (pyelonephritis) generally begins in your urethra or bladder and travels to one or both of your kidneys. Bacteria that enter your urinary tract through the tube that carries urine from your body (urethra) can multiply and travel to your kidneys. This is the most common cause of kidney infections... A kidney infection requires prompt medical attention. If not treated properly, a kidney infection can permanently damage your kidneys or can cause a life-threatening infection.[195]

Reduce risk of kidney infection by taking steps to prevent urinary tract infections. They don't always cause signs and symptoms, but when they do they may include: A strong, persistent urge to urinate; A burning sensation when urinating; Passing frequent, small amounts of urine; Urine that appears cloudy; Urine that appears red, bright pink or cola-colored — a sign of blood in the urine; Strong-smelling urine; Pelvic pain, in women — especially in the center of the pelvis and around the area of the pubic bone.[193]

Interstitial cystitis and urethritis

Interstitial Cystitis is a chronic condition causing bladder pressure, bladder pain and sometimes pelvic pain. The pain ranges from mild discomfort to severe. Your bladder is a hollow, muscular organ that stores urine. The bladder expands until it's full and then signals your brain that it's time to urinate. With interstitial cystitis, these signals get mixed up — you feel the need to urinate more often and with smaller volumes of urine than most people. Interstitial cystitis most often affects women and can have a long-lasting impact on quality of life. Although there's no cure, medications and other therapies may offer relief.[196]

Urethritis is inflammation (swelling and irritation) of the tube that carries urine from the body. Both bacteria and viruses may cause urethritis. Some of the bacteria that cause this condition include E coli, chlamydia, and gonorrhea. These bacteria also cause urinary tract infections and some sexually transmitted diseases. Viral causes are herpes simplex virus and cytomegalovirus.[197]

During sex, bacteria can be driven up the urine tube to cause infection. A simple "rinsing" of the opening with fresh and soothing water before and after sex may reduce this risk, and leave you feeling cleansed and comfortable as well. Nearly any bidet is an excellent way to keep your genital areas clean, providing a non-irritating, thorough cleansing with fresh water and an adjustable spray. Bidets also eliminate the need for most deodorant sprays or feminine products such as douches, a clear benefit in light of the fact that chemical irritation from products like these are another known risk factor for urinary tract infections.

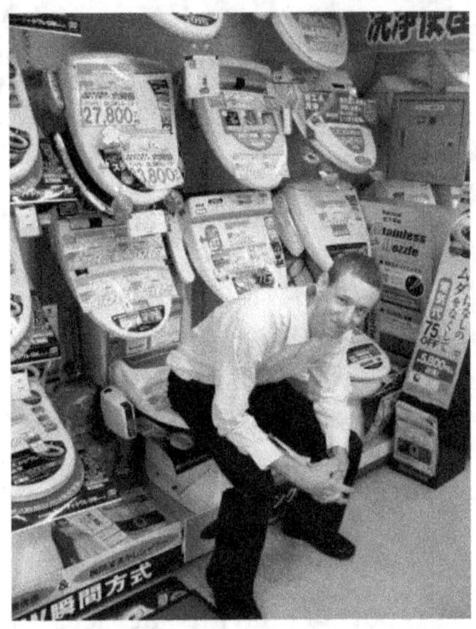

Bowel Dysfunction

Oddly, all I had to do was either use a bidet (that I don't have) or hop in the shower and rinse it off after. I was told specifically not to use soap or rub at it with TP. It's kind of a moot point because the oxy or percocet cause such extreme constipation that I couldn't poop for over a week (can't remember which but both are narcotics so it's the same result).[308]

Anal fissure is one of the most common causes of severe anal pain. Factors which predispose people to develop anal fissure include diarrhea, constipation, childbirth, medication as well as constant saddle vibration (amongst professional mountain-bikers) and using a [strong, single] jet of water from a bidet-toilet.[309]

Constipation and Diarrhea

Constipation is a common symptom affecting between 2 percent and 27 percent of the population in Western countries. In the United States, it results in more than 2.5 million visits to physicians, 92,000 hospitalizations, and laxative sales of several hundred million dollars a year. Constipation is more prevalent in women than in men, in nonwhites than in white persons, in children than in adults, and in elderly than in younger adults. Severe constipation (e.g., bowel movements only twice a month) is seen almost exclusively in women. Physical inactivity, low income, limited education, a history of sexual abuse, and symptoms of depression are all risk factors for constipation.[7]

Bowel habits are a difficult function to study objectively because of their highly private nature and negative associations. Therefore, it is not surprising that they represent one of the least understood aspects of human behavior... Prospective studies on bowel habits conducted over an adequate period of time in the general population are still lacking.[144]

Many health authorities believe that constipation is the number one affliction underlying nearly every ailment... This means that constipation would be the most prevalent ailment affecting the civilized world... It is vital to stress that constipation affects the health of the colon, upon which the health of the body in its entirety depends.[277]

People have died from pooping too hard. It caused their blood pressure to rise enough to shake loose a blood clot or burst an aneurysm.[297]

Almost all functions of the gastrointestinal tract have been shown to be under central nervous control and to respond to environmental factors such as stress. It is, therefore, not surprising that disturbed gastrointestinal functions (including defecation) may be altered through psychological therapy... Psychological management usually consisted of relaxation training, stress management and patient information. Additional behavioral modification, e.g. of eating and defecation behavior, is superior to pharmacological and dietary management alone.[145]

In another study 69% reported having at least one of 20 functional gastrointestinal syndromes in the previous three months. The symptoms were attributed to four major anatomic regions: esophageal (42%), gastroduodenal (26%), bowel (44%), and anorectal (26%), with considerable overlap.[146] In a study of young adults, "Only 3.6% of subjects reported diarrhea greater than 25% of the time, and only 7.3% reported constipation greater than 25% of the time".[147] (Yet this adds up to about 11% of our population with a reported bowel dysfunction greater than 25% of the time.)

Patients with spinal cord injury used an electronic bidet with an imaging device to facilitate precise hitting of the anal area with water streams to stimulate bowel movement. Bowel movement was successfully induced in 15 of the 20 patients (75%). Success was not related significantly to injury level, or ability to voluntarily squeeze. Compared with their usual manner of bowel management, for which they spent more than 30 minutes, time needed for successful bowel movement was shortened in 11 of 13 patients. No complications were observed.[148]

Elvis biographer Joel Williamson writes, "For some reason — perhaps involving a reaction to the codeine and attempts to move his bowels — he experienced pain and fright while sitting on the toilet. Alarmed, he stood up, dropped the book he was reading, stumbled forward, and fell face down in the fetal position. He struggled weakly and drooled on the rug. Unable to breathe, he died."[26] This led to the common saying, "The King died on the throne". -- John Voelz, King Me (Littleton, CO 2010)[312]

Constipation

The expression constipation is derived from the Latin word "constiatus" which translated means to press or crowd together, to pack, to cram. Consequently, to be constipated means that the packed accumulation of feces in the bowel makes its evacuation difficult.[277]   Constipation and defecation may be considered as the last taboo. The inability of defecate or to achieve this only by digital evacuation (digging it out with your finger) has never been a popular topic among patients and doctors.[49] Chronic constipation is one of the most prevalent gastrointestinal conditions presenting to primary care physicians globally that severely impacts the quality of life of those affected. Prevalence of chronic constipation (in the U.S.) is 15.0–19.9%.[150]

Many health authorities believe that constipation is the number one affliction underlying nearly every ailment. This means that constipation would be the most prevalent ailment affecting the civilized world. It is vital to stress that constipation affects the health of the colon, upon which the health of the body in its entirety depends. Constipation contributes toward the lowering of body resistance predisposing it to many acute illnesses and the creation of a great many degenerative and chronic processes. Almost every human ailment has been attributed to a malfunctioning colon, i.e., one that cannot perform its normal, regular and efficient functioning.[277]

Although chronic constipation is a common symptom, to date no international consensus has been reached regarding its definition... In the internet survey, 28.4% of the respondents considered themselves to be constipated. Stratified by sex, significantly more females (37.5%) than males (19.1%) considered themselves to be constipated... Increased water intake was the most commonly held idea as a countermeasure against constipation (52.2%, 2693/5155 respondents). The next most common idea was to get more sleep (39.7%), followed by changes in diet (38.6%), use of a bidet-toilet (37.1%), reduction of stress (31.0%), and exercise (25.3%).[152]

The primary symptom which elderly people used to define constipation was having to strain in order to defecate. Multiple factors were found to influence self-reports of constipation... The number of chronic illnesses and the number of no laxative medications were significantly related to constipation in women but not men.[153]

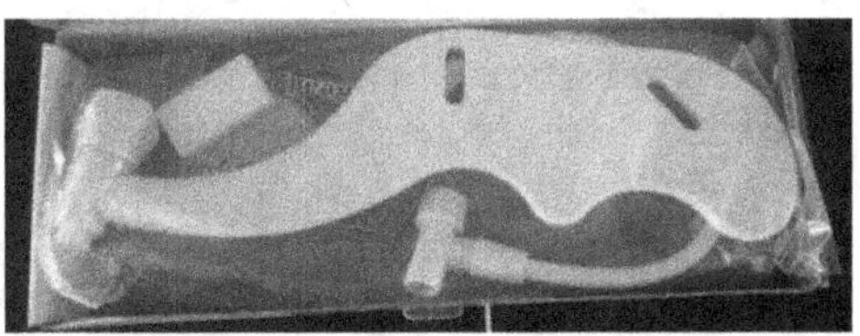

Constipation is a common condition occurring with increasing frequency in advanced age. As a symptom, it is not always dealt with directly by the physician, but is often left to the care of nurses. Many patients rely on self-medication. Constipation not only interferes with the quality of life, often it requires competent medical intervention. Constipation is a condition of clinical importance.[218]

A Korean study that investigated factors influencing constipation in school age children (4-6 grade) found that Bidet users had a much lower incidence of constipation (11.8%) than seat toilets (62.4%) and Squat toilets (25.8%). While stress had the highest correlation with constipation, there were some telling attitudes towards standard school toilets: "It is common that there isn't any toilet paper... I am hesitate to sit on the toilet... I feel uncomfortable when I sit on the toilet... I cannot concentrate if I defecate in the school toilet... The toilet makes me feel dirty".[154]

There are good arguments that most forms of constipation have psychological and/or neurological components. Research has demonstrated that approximately half of those suffering from chronic constipation do not have a physical ailment; their constipation comes from nervous or psychological causes that prevent the relaxation of the sphincters (anal valves).[145,154-55] The gentle spray from the bidet provides a form of hydro-massage that has been shown to help this condition. Read more on this in **Hydro-Massage, Hydrotherapy, etc.**

Fantastic product, Great features and quality... I feel it is important to mention that this unit comes with two types of rear washes. One is a "regular" rear cleaning which is a more direct water stream, and the other is a soft rear, which fans the water out slightly more than the regular rear cleaning. Both can have oscillation enabled at the touch of a button, and the nozzle can easily be adjusted forward or backward depending on your body type. The regular rear cleaning, combined with the oscillation is the one that can help those with constipation issues. Both the soft and regular give a solid clean, but I feel it worth mentioning in case anyone needs it for this purpose.[1]

Stress and Dysfunction

Half the patients that suffer from chronic constipation have what is called dyssynergic defecation. Essentially this is failure of co-ordination, the inability to relax the rectal and anal muscles that allow a stool to exit. This is thought to be a behavioral disorder.[155]

Constipation is a symptom complex and not merely a disease. In the absence of secondary causes, it is due to either a neuromuscular dysfunction of the colon—slow transit constipation—or a neuromuscular dysfunction of the defecation unit. In many patients, there is an overlap because colon transit is delayed in two thirds of patients with difficult or disordered defecation. Studies have shown that most patients with difficult defecation show a failure of rectoanal coordination that consists of impaired abdominal and rectal pushing forces, or paradoxic anal contraction or inadequate anal relaxation. A lack of coordination or dyssynergia of the abdominal and pelvic floor muscles that are involved in defecation appears to be the primary underlying mechanism.[155]

Neuromuscular conditioning using biofeedback techniques is a useful method of treatment for patients with refractory defecation disorders such as fecal incontinence or constipation with obstructive defecation. In patients with obstructive defecation, the goals are to relax the anal sphincter, improve rectoanal coordination, and improve sensory perception. After biofeedback therapy, symptomatic improvement has been reported in 70 to 80% of patients with either incontinence or obstructive defecation. Recent studies also demonstrated objective improvement in anorectal function.[75]

Studies have found that up to 78% of constipated children close the anal canal while straining by contracting the anal sphincter. This paradoxical anal closure was thought to be the result of a self-conditioning process by the children. When treated with biofeedback therapy, most children were successfully re-conditioned to relax their anal sphincter during defecation, which helped to relieve them from constipation and soiling.[75-6]

Twelve children with paradoxical anal closure were treated by biofeedback therapy. The results showed that all these children were successfully conditioned to relax their anal sphincter during defecation. This therapy improved their bowel habits and relieved them from constipation and soiling. The results proposed that the paradoxical anal closure itself is the result of a self-conditioning process. In this process, the patient learns to paradoxically contract the external anal sphincter in response to the urge and the act of defecation. Biofeedback therapy seems to be the appropriate treatment in such cases.[76]

Constipated adults may also paradoxically increase anal resistance by straining. In one study of severely constipated young women, all failed to relax their external anal sphincter (EAS) on attempted defecation, and 80% of these patients actually contracted their EAS when they strained to defecate, causing a functional outlet obstruction.[162] In another study, 30 of 31 constipated patients exhibited this pattern, and 20% of the "healthy" controls also closed the anal canal while trying to defecate.[163]

Psychological distress levels did not seem to be important in explaining GI symptom change over a 1-yr period in one study. Psychological distress, however, was linked to having persistent GI symptoms and frequently seeking health care for them over time. Perhaps clinicians should consider psychological factors in the treatment of this subset of irritable bowel syndrome patients.[158]

Contrary to current dogma, psycho-social factors were significantly associated with functional GI disorders in this community sample.[159]

In one rural outpatient primary care population, functional impairment was explained more by psychological distress than by severity of medical illness. Decreasing the burden of psychological distress among primary care patients seemed to improve functioning.[160]

High rates of psychiatric disorder have been documented in patients with functional bowel syndromes. Individuals with two or more medically unexplained gastrointestinal symptoms had high rates of psychiatric disorders.[161]

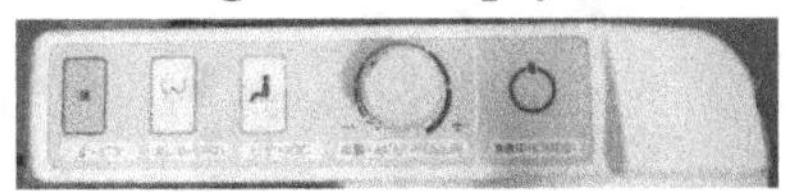

Blowing up a balloon in the rectum and the onset of pain were perceived in constipated patients at volumes that were not significantly different from those in normal volunteers. Constipated patients, however, required higher rectal volumes to induce the desire to defecate and to stimulate regular rectal contractions. Constipated patients also found it more difficult to pass simulated stools from the rectum than the normal controls and, unlike most normal controls, failed to relax their external anal sphincter on attempted defecation.[165]

Neuromuscular conditioning (habit retraining) is an instrument-based learning technique. Seventy to eighty percent of patients gain symptomatic improvement through biofeedback.[75] Additionally, biofeedback is effective in teaching relaxation of anal muscles in many anorectal disorders, and can recondition and improve bowel function.[75-76]

I personally, and a number of bidet manufacturers as well, report that the massaging effect of the spray helps relax the anal sphincters making defecation easier, not unlike the biofeedback described above. They recommend a bidet as a simple and safe instrument that might be of value for anyone who suffers from constipation. An electronic bidet that provides warm (38 °C) water and very low force (10 mN) with a fountain type of flow, will lower anal resting pressure essentially the same amount as a sitz bath.[133]

Lack of Stimulation

Unlike your skin, the rectum has no ability to feel pain, heat, or other sensations, but is quite sensitive to swelling from internal pressure.[166]

Three sensory thresholds are usually defined: constant sensation of fullness, urge to defecate, and maximum tolerated volume.[166] Finally, in this group we can find those patients having the so-called fecal impaction, that is an abnormality of either sensitivity or stimulus to defecate frequently observed in the elderly and in children.[167]

Many who are constipated need more internal pressure than others (which usually means higher rectal volumes) to get their bodies to defecate. Rectal contractions, anal relaxation and a desire to defecate all require more pressure.[165,168] How much more volume is needed? In one study, 60 ml fluid injected into the rectum was enough to induce defecation.[169] (60 ml equals about 2 fluid ounces, 1/4 cup, or 4 tablespoons).

Subjects perceived a rectal sensation within one second of rapid inflation of a rectal balloon with volumes of 20 ml or less air. Six patients did not perceive any rectal sensation until 60 ml had been introduced, while in the remaining nine patients the sensation was delayed by at least two seconds.[169]

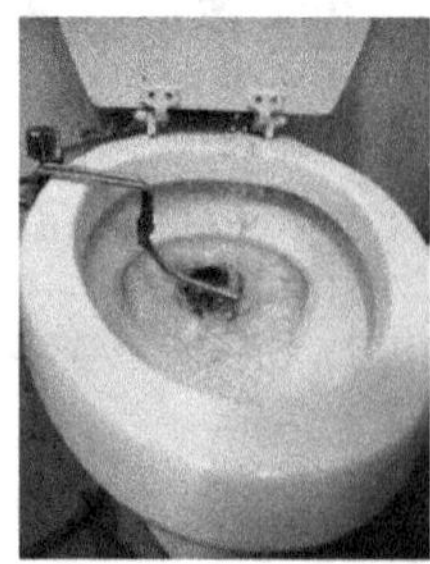

Although the primary use of the electronic bidet was to clean the anus after toileting and wash the perineal area, many additional functions have been developed to improve our convenience. These days the water pressure and water temperature can be selected by the user, and the water jet angle can be varied from narrow to wide. A high-pressure water jet flow is now provided by some of the manufacturers to aid defecation. One study investigated whether water pressures in these jets are higher than resting anal sphincter pressure, and whether water might penetrate into the rectum and stimulate defecation. By measuring increases in rectal temperature after applying warm water, researchers were able to confirm that this is the case, concluding that if water ingress exceeds this capacity, rectal pressures could elevate and promote defecation. It is possible that the bidet defecatory function might be somewhat poorer than an enema in terms of evoking anal sphincter contractions, although most bidet users considered it to be considerably more convenient.[170]

[2016] Seventy-nine (230) individuals were using the warm-water washing toilet seat. There was no significant difference in age between the usage group and the non-use group. The purposes of use after defection, for defecation induction, and after urination and for washing the vagina were 90.4, 41.3, and 40.4%, respectively. Regarding the kinds of washing, a strong tendency for the use of the anal washing function to induce defection and after defection was observed, whereas a tendency was observed for the use of the bidet function after urination and for washing the vagina. Many individuals were using the washing function for the purpose of inducing defection and after urination.[206]

For me personally, when I cannot easily defecate, if I inject a little water into my rectum with my bidet, I get a full bowel movement within seconds. My successful experiences with this approach is described in the **Appendix**.

Hemorrhoids

Hemorrhoids are swollen veins in your anus and lower rectum, similar to varicose veins. The veins around your anus tend to stretch under pressure and may bulge or swell. Swollen veins (hemorrhoids) can develop from increased pressure in the lower rectum. Hemorrhoids are more likely with older adults because the tissues that support the veins in your rectum and anus can thin, weaken and stretch.[184]

Hemorrhoids have plagued humankind since time immemorial, yet many misunderstandings regarding hemorrhoid complaints and disease still exist. The risk of getting hemorrhoids increases with straining to defecate, constipation, low dietary fiber intake, pregnancy and delivery, obesity, diarrhea, anal infection, and certain occupations that require continual standing or sitting.[236]

Hemorrhoids bother about 89% of all Americans at some time in their lives. Hemorrhoids caused Napoleon to sit side-saddle, sent President Jimmy Carter to the operating room, and benched baseball star George Brett during the 1980 World Series. Physical examinations have revealed that over two thirds of all healthy people have hemorrhoids.[186]

Symptoms of external hemorrhoids can be: Itching or irritation in your anal region; perianal pain or discomfort; swelling around your anus; or bleeding. You usually can't see or feel internal hemorrhoids, but straining or irritation when passing stool can cause painless bleeding during bowel movements. A hemorrhoid can be pushed through the anal opening resulting in pain and irritation. Thrombosed hemorrhoids are an external hemorrhoid that forms a blood clot (thrombus), it can result in severe pain, swelling, inflammation or a hard lump near your anus.[236]

The Travel Bidet is great! I don't know how I ever lived without it! My excess weight has always been a problem in cleaning myself properly. Now that I have a bidet I am clean and I no longer have vaginal infections nor do I have bleeding hemorrhoids.[9]

Stabilization of Hemorrhoids

For people who suffer from hemorrhoids, as I have for years, this is a must. Using toilet paper and even pre-moistened wipes are abrasive and can aggravate an already painful situation. Your bidet provides an easy, efficient and painless way to better hygiene. I highly recommend [bidets] to everyone. If you suffer from discomfort this will dramatically improve your comfort level. If you don't, it will help you improve your personal hygiene, make you feel fresher, and help you avoid possible future problems. Dr. Greg Lousignont.[164]

A bidet can offer benefits if you suffer from hemorrhoids. Because of the swelling and irritation that comes from wiping with toilet paper even using light pressure on the affected area may be excruciating. This often causes you to wipe ineffectively, leaving behind residue that leaves you feeling unclean and that can lead to infection in some cases.

The water from the bidet will cool your inflamed hemorrhoids while also cleaning your anal area completely. Since you do not wipe you will not add further inflammation and irritation to your already sore behind. Using water can also eliminate rectal itching that can be caused when you are not cleaning your anal area properly because of discomfort.[187]

EXCESSIVE CLEANSING of the anal area with soap and water can cause big problems if you are suffering with prolapsing internal hemorrhoids or external hemorrhoids. You remove natural oils from the skin surface in the area and increase friction when you move, walk, etc. THE AREA MUST BE KEPT LUBRICATED! THIS IS OF UTMOST IMPORTANCE!!!... Regular (the cheaper the worse) toilet paper might be regarded as very fine sand paper. Do you really want that for YOUR delicate hemorrhoids ? If possible, wash yourself and DAB dry, don't WIPE... Also, consider use of a bidet. There are many web sites on the use of this cleansing method unfamiliar to many Americans, but potentially very useful for those suffering from hemorrhoids.[124]

Straining and constipation have long been thought of as culprits in the formation of hemorrhoids, so first-line treatment for all first- and second-degree internal hemorrhoids should include measures to decrease straining and constipation. Bidets are excellent for this.[184-89] Anything that speeds up the defecation process is of benefit. This has been covered in the previous section **Bowel Dysfunction**.

58

In one prospective 1-year follow-up study of bidet toilet users, researchers found that hemorrhoids and urogenital infections, excluding bacterial vaginitis, were not causally related to habitual bidet toilet use.[189]

Reddit website - This is a fabulous product. Why didn't I have this before? I have never felt so clean. I was never happy with just toilet paper & have been spending a small fortune on wipes for years. Now one wipe is all I need.[190]

I bought a bidet 3 months ago and haven't pooped anywhere else since... until today. Sometimes when I wipe... I'll wipe and I'll wipe and I'll wipe and I'll wipe... a hundred times. Still poop, still poop. It's like I'm wiping a marker or something.[190]

There is clearly a potential for allergic reactions to components of moist toilet paper and reactions to recycled toilet paper presumably irritant by nature [including likely presence of dioxins]. These irritant reactions are probably caused by the rough texture of current paper types and do not reflect the presence of potentially toxic ingredients such as metal salts.[85]

Diarrhea and Incontinence
Leaking loose, watery stools

Bidets can greatly aid neuromuscular conditioning to control diarrhea and/or incontinence as a biofeedback device. Neuromuscular conditioning using biofeedback techniques is a useful method of treatment for patients with refractory defecation disorders such as fecal incontinence or constipation with obstructive defecation. In patients with incontinence, the goals are to improve the strength of the anal sphincter, improve sensory perception, and improve coordination between the rectum and anal sphincter. After biofeedback therapy, symptomatic improvement has been reported in 70 to 80% of patients with either incontinence or obstructive defecation. Recent studies also demonstrated objective improvement in anorectal function.[75] Bidets are biofeedback devices.

Diarrhea

Diarrhea is the condition of having at least three loose, liquid, or watery bowel movements each day. It often lasts for a few days and can result in dehydration due to fluid loss.[157]

Diarrhea necessitates constant trips to the toilet, with the subsequent need to constantly wipe the anus dry. The friction caused by constant rubbing with toilet paper can cause severe irritation and chafing of the skin. This can be especially painful for young children. Worse yet, some diarrhea can cause children to excrete fluid discharges that are significantly acidic, further adding to the inflammation, pain and general discomfort.[171]

Lactose intolerance is a condition in which people have symptoms due to the decreased ability to digest lactose, a sugar found in dairy products. Those affected vary in the amount of lactose they can tolerate before symptoms develop. Symptoms may include abdominal pain, bloating, diarrhea, gas, and nausea.[172].... and diarrhea from personal experience.

The cleansing nozzles of bidets can easily and frequently flush away these bodily fluids, while the natural buffering of the water minimizes any irritating acidity. Some bidets will also air dry the area after use, obviating any need for further physical touch or rubbing.

Diaper Rash: Infants are very prone to this. The acid in the diarrhea can literally burn your child's sensitive skin. This is also prime smelly diaper time. What can you do to to prevent some of these worst moments as a parent? The best way is preventative - by applying a thick layer of ointment over and around their bottom to protect the skin before the rash starts. Instead of rubbing the skin with a standard wipe consider washing it gently with mild soap and water or to use a bidet to gently wash the skin to prevent further irritation.[171]

Incontinence

Fecal incontinence is the inability to control your bowel movements, causing stool (feces) to leak unexpectedly from your rectum. Also called bowel incontinence, fecal incontinence can range from an occasional leakage of stool while passing gas to a complete loss of bowel control. Common causes of fecal incontinence include diarrhea, constipation, and muscle or nerve damage... Skin irritation. The skin around the anus is delicate and sensitive. Repeated contact with stool can lead to pain and itching, and potentially to sores (ulcers) that require medical treatment. Avoid straining. Straining during bowel movements can eventually weaken anal sphincter muscles or damage nerves, possibly leading to fecal incontinence.[173]

The social and psychological consequences of incontinence are serious. Incontinent elderly view their condition as a significant symbol of loss of control as well as self-esteem, and is discussed by them in terms of infantilization. It is regarded as a risk to their independent status, and frequently results in becoming house-bound, withdrawn, and socially isolated. There may also be a decline in personal care, nutritional status, and physical health. Also the prevalence of anxiety and depression is five times as great in incontinent elderly people. Urinary incontinence is seen as one of several factors contributing to caregiver "breaking point" and the related decision to seek nursing home care.[175]

Self-reported fecal incontinence, defined as involuntary loss of anal sphincteric control leading to unwanted release of liquid or solid feces at an inappropriate time or in an inappropriate place, within the past 12 months. The response rate was 66%. The prevalence of solid or liquid fecal incontinence was 2% and 9%, respectively. The mean age of subjects with fecal incontinence was 53 years; 55% were women. Despite significant associated morbidity, most cases of fecal incontinence were unrecognized by doctors.[176]

The cost of incontinence in U.S. nursing homes has been calculated at $2 billion dollars annually, while the costs associated with outpatient management of the problem in the community setting are estimated to be about $6 billion per year. Collectively, these figures represent an enormous financial drain on the U.S. health-care system.[175]

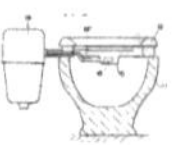

We do know that to prevent perineal skin injury, it is helpful to prevent excessive skin hydration, minimize the interaction of urine and feces, minimize local microorganisms, and maintain skin near its physiologic pH.[135]

Treating Incontinence

Fecal Incontinence is a debilitating, embarrassing, and potentially devastating disorder. It is common and affects up to 24% of the general population, although figures vary widely depending on the definition of fecal incontinence and the age group studied. The prevalence of fecal incontinence is even higher in institutionalized and nursing home patients. Complaints of fecal incontinence can range from fatal incontinence to minor soiling with small amounts of liquid stool or stool pellets to frank, involuntary passage of a complete bowel movement.[185]

Change their diaper frequently. Instead of rubbing the skin with a standard wipe consider washing them gently with mild soap and water to prevent further irritation.[171]

Aging skin experiences increased dryness allowing cracks in which bacteria colonizes and slower recovery from the effects of alkaline substances. Skin should be cleansed gently without high alkalinity (as in some bar soaps) or rubbing (which denudes fragile skin). Aged skin should be patted or air dried, moisturized after bathing, and protected with a barrier.[143]

Bidets allow multiple washings without increased skin abrasion or irritation. For those suffering from incontinence travel bidets may be a godsend. Amazingly compact, they can allow sufferers to pursue their daily lives knowing that they can at least wash away the results without having to resort to rubbing with toilet paper. Many people who suffer from incontinence benefit from biofeedback training.

Biofeedback is extensively used in clinical practice to treat fecal incontinence... Of those studies with adequate data, 275 out of 566 patients (49%) were said to be cured of symptoms of fecal incontinence following biofeedback therapy and 617 out of 861(72%) patients were reported to be cured or improved.[281]

After biofeedback therapy, symptomatic improvement has been reported in 70 to 80% of patients with either incontinence or obstructive defecation. Recent studies also demonstrated objective improvement in anorectal function.[75]

In the previous section on constipation I presented an argument that bidets could replicate much of the positive effects of biofeedback. While I have no great experience with incontinence, it seems likely that regular use of bidets could have a similar positive effect in such training.

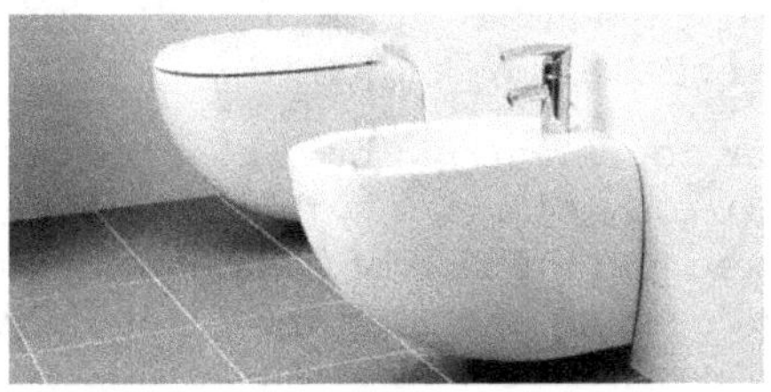

Hydro-Massage, Hydrotherapy, Hydropathy

The use of water for pain relief and treatment.[282]

Hydrotherapy is the use of water to treat a disease or to maintain health. The theory behind it is that water has many properties that give it the ability to heal: Water can store and carry heat and energy; Water can dissolve other substances, such as minerals and salts; Water cannot hurt you, even if you are sensitive to your surroundings... Water can help blood flow. Water has a soothing, calming, and relaxing effect on people, whether in a bath, shower, spray, or compress... People use hydrotherapy to treat many illnesses and conditions, including acne; arthritis; colds; depression; headaches; stomach problems; joint, muscle, and nerve problems; sleep disorders; and stress. People also use it for relaxation and to maintain health. You can also use hydrotherapy to reduce or relieve sudden or long-lasting pain... Hydrotherapy is generally safe if treatment is done properly.[179]

People have always been naturally drawn to water as a source of comfort—the soothing sounds of a bubbling brook, the relaxing steam of a natural hot spring, or just a good evening soak. Some of the best calming features of water are opening our blood vessels to improve circulation and relaxing our muscles; thus providing an escape from the pressures of daily life.

Hydro massage gently warms and stimulates the muscles and joints, expediting recovery to the benefit of those with injuries and muscle pain. It reduces pain levels in those with arthritis by opening the blood vessels and increasing range of movement, and reduces muscle tension and overall discomfort resulting from fibromyalgia. And for those who suffer from lower-back pain, a 2012 article in the **Journal of Musculoskeletal Research** found that hydrotherapy provides more potential benefits when compared to land-based exercises.[284]

If you look up hydro-massage on Google or other search sites on the web you will find that every luxury hotel and spa offers it in some form and claims therapeutic benefits. Massage schools and other alternative health schools teach a variety of hydro-massage techniques (hydrotherapy, Hydrotherapy Showers, whirlpool, watsu-aqua shiatsu, etc.). Some medical plans even cover hydrotherapy as useful medical treatment.[179]

Jacuzzi and other forms of whirlpool baths have sold millions of units to satisfied customers. Everyone I know has enjoyed a hot tub experience with Jacuzzi jets. When I have abused muscles, a hot shower with lots of pressure is definitely beneficial.

The National Institutes of Health estimates that 30 percent of Americans suffer from sleep disruption. All the benefits of immersing yourself in warm water—tension relief, improved circulation and more—also help create healthy sleep habits, according to the Better Sleep Council.[284]

Hallo everybody ! Your conversation about bidet is very interesting to me! I am from Italy and I have to say I find it highly higenic. After living in England for some years, I realised that the rate of female genitalia diseases due to less higenic conditions (like cystitis) much higher that in Italy.[12]

Perianal Hydro-massage

While you are washing off with the bidet spray, you also are receiving a certain amount of stimulation, or hydro-massage, from using the bidet. Hydro-massage has always been considered therapeutic. When I wrote the First Edition it was a long search to find anyone who had studied the medical benefits of hydro-massage on any skin (epithelium) anywhere on the body.

This might be an unpleasant similie, but gingiva in your mouth is also epithelium, is also mucous membrane, and its mucous nature is not unlike the tender interior epithelium of your colon (sorry, but true). Both are exceedingly difficult areas to keep the skin healthy. If you can accept this comparison, research on gum disease may shed some light on the area of perianal/genital health.

Stimulation of gums with a pulsating water jet irrigator improved chronic inflammatory periodontal disease. It showed statistically highly significant improvements in plaque index, gingival index, succubus bleeding index, gingival shrinkage and probable pocket depth.[285] In one classic study, local lymphization and lymph transport were stimulated, following manual massage of tissues. Lymph levels of protein and lymphocytes rose.[286]

We have cited studies that say tap water is just fine for irritated tissue and wounds. Here is another slightly more extreme test of tap water. More striking is the next study of post-operative washing. Even within hours of sugary, water cleansing is fine.

Acute traumatic soft tissue wounds were cleaned with tap water and sterile saline. The infection rate in wounds cleaned with sterile saline was 10.3% but only 5.4% in wounds cleaned with tap water. There were no microbiological differences between the two groups.[287] Bidets of course make a fine source of tap water for cleaning.

The evidence reviewed suggests that early bathing or showering of surgical wound incisions does not pose a risk of infection. Patients can return to their normal bathing or showering routine as soon as 12 hours after surgery and, perhaps even earlier, without the fear of increasing their risk of infection. We found no data discussing evidenced-based reasons for keeping a wound dry and covered until suture removal.[288]

Massage, irrigation, stimulation, whatever you call it, improves skin health, and the water massage of a bidet does this very gently.

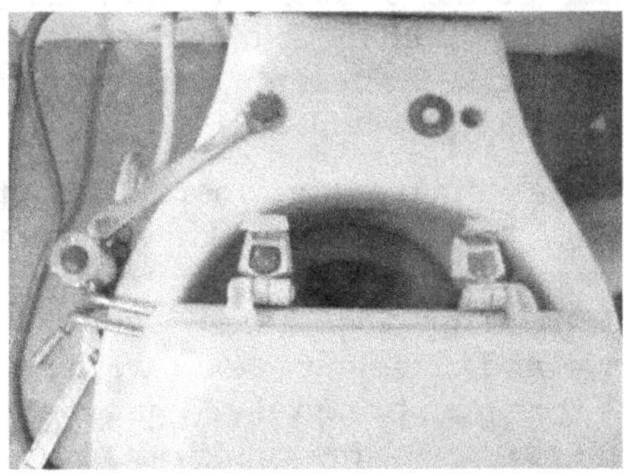

[2010] I was unable to find a single controlled clinical trial to substantiate the claims... it seems fair to say that the therapeutic claims made by professional organizations of colonic irrigation are unsubstantiated. A recent survey suggested that colonic irrigation is totally devoid of risks: during 8470 treatments... no adverse events were noted.[283]

Sixteen patients suffered from fecal soiling (Group I), whereas the other 16 patients were treated for fecal incontinence (Group II). Patients were instructed by enterostomal therapists how to use a conventional colostomy irrigation set to obtain sufficient irrigation of the distal part of their large bowel... In Group I, irrigation was found to be beneficial in 92 percent of patients, whereas 60 percent of patients in Group II considered the treatment as a major improvement to the quality of their lives... it might be worthwhile to treat these patients first by colonic irrigation.[181]

Colonic irrigation with ACIA is safe and can improve abdominal pain, constipation, and diarrhea associated with irritable bowel syndrome (IBS). Patients were more satisfied with their bowel movements and found their symptoms were less disturbing.[290]

Fifteen years ago I could find no peer-reviewed medical research to substantiate the medical value of colon hydrotherapy. Nevertheless I have been practicing a version of this since before publishing the first edition of this book with significant health benefits. See **Appendix**.

Colon hydrotherapy is the safe, gentle infusion of purified warm water into the colon under conditions that offer safety, using no chemicals or drugs. It is the natural solution to conditions which interfere with the normal functions of the colon... To be in optimum health the colon must be functioning normally... I believe that the colon is one of the most neglected areas by the medical establishment. One of the major indications for colon hydrotherapy is constipation... In our clinic we find that people with all kinds of skin problems (i.e., acne, psoriasis, eczema, etc.) usually can benefit from a therapeutic course of colon irrigations. The skin is the largest excretory organ in the body. When the colon is sluggish or clogged up or there are a lot of toxins in the body, the skin may act as a major excretory organ. Unhealthy skin is usually a sign of an unhealthy colon and no amount of antibiotics, skin creams or medications will alleviate the problems until the cause of the problem is addressed... Almost every human ailment has been attributed to a malfunctioning colon (i.e., one that cannot perform its normal, regular and efficient functioning) - Donald J. Mantell, M.D.[277]

I am not from the USA or a Latin country, where the people seems to believe toilet paper is unhygienic. In all my 53 years I have done well with toilet paper thank you. Bidets are rare in South Africa too. However, over the last 2 years I developed a condition where my bowels are not working properly and I need frequent trips to the loo and sometimes need washing not only in the butt crack but even into the rectum to bring relief. I just returned from a hotel with a bidet and found it very handy with the aim to install one at home.[216]

Bidets and Anal Cleansing

Below are the positions of two bidet manufacturers on anal cleansing with the bidet. I personally have used my handheld bidet to induce defecation for at least 14 years. Read more about this in the **Appendix**.

This is the way I use the Hygeia (bidet) — 1. My Hygeia is permanently installed by the water closet so that the spray unit can be placed under the toilet seat. 2. The water valve at the spray unit is in the off position and the cold water is turned on. 3. When I sit down the spray unit can be moved to the center of the anal area. 4. The special designed spray is slowly turned on for the water to magically enter the rectum. There are eight jets that apexes at the anal orifice. 5. When I feel enough water has entered the rectum I turn the water valve off and let nature do her thing. 6. Here now is the key to a happy fanny, always there is feces remaining in the rectum so I repeat the flushing for complete removal. I know this is why I feel like a million dollars the rest of the day. I sit with a comfort I cannot explain, I walk with a spring in my step, and I play golf with a more fluid movement. All sportsmen would have an edge if they regularly used this unit. I know doctors that are excited in using it. For various reasons, no tightening of the buttocks... I use the Jennings Hygeia less than two minutes for my bowel defecation. Shower fresh, yes, but double fresh for the remaining feces in the rectum is flushed out in final cleaning. - Wayne Jennings [164]

The upward stream of water, provided by the bidet, directly into the rectum in a steady stream serves to relax the internal and external sphincter muscles controlling the anus, thus permitting contraction of the muscular walls of the rectum, causing feces to be more easily passed without straining. The bidet's cleansing nozzle stimulates a bowel movement by relaxing the sphincters and lubricating the anus. A 8-10 second application of direct warm water flow is recommended prior to attempting to defecate. Increasing the water pressure with the pressure control valve allows the water to penetrate much in the same way as an enema and brings about a gentle, comfortable, more natural elimination. Daily use of the Bidet for this purpose gradually teaches the user how to relax thus relieving constipation through a natural habit. [183]

The tap water tested was generally agreed to be safe from harmful bacteria and had no contaminating bacteria; Human and rat models showed a clear benefit in using tap water to cleanse soft tissue wounds, thus concluding tap water is safe for use on wounds. [37]

Your colon is very important to you, and life-threatening if it is stupidly misused. You should only try anal cleansing under the supervision of an experienced health provider, at least at first.

Your ass is super absorptive, which is why chugging beer, wine, or hard liquor from your ass ("butt chugging") is super dangerous. Without running alcohol through your liver and kidneys first, you lose the ability to puke when you've had way too much. This means you can easily butt chug too much and die. Don't try it at home, kids! [297]

Rectal or vaginal surgery traumatizes the skin.[202] A soft spray or mist from a bidet can both soothe and wash the area for optimum healing. The benefits of a simple water spray on irritated or damaged skin have been discussed in previous sections.[93-6] Below are three more studies on the effectiveness of a water jet in healing surgical wounds.

The purpose of this study was to determine if hydro debridement with pulsed lavage facilitates the removal of necrotic tissue, promotes healing, and increases comfort in the homebound patient. Home healthcare provides cost-effective care in the setting that is most conducive to healing. People want to be at home, yet many illnesses require services that cannot be obtained at home... All of the clients in the sample achieved a clean, warm, moist wound bed, free of signs and symptoms of infection, absence of necrotic tissue, and the presence of granulation tissue to meet the definition of "ready for healing" as presented in the literature. The majority of clients experienced no pain. Although comorbid conditions required re-hospitalization for 35.7% of the sample, the conditions did not interfere with healing. Hydrodebridement with pulsed lavage is a viable no traumatic, noninvasive, site-specific treatment alternative for patients receiving care in the home.[210]

Thorough irrigation of contaminated or infected traumatic and open surgical wounds is considered standard practice. High-power pulse lavage (40 psi) is frequently used to facilitate the removal of surface contaminants and bacteria but studies to compare the results of various irrigation techniques are limited... The results of this study confirm that cleansing contaminated or infected acute wounds using high pressure (at least 15 psi) reduces wound bacterial counts. Studies to compare the clinical outcomes of various irrigation techniques and pressure ranges are warranted and the potential benefit of selective debridement using the high-pressure parallel water jet should be investigated.[211]

The aim was to assess the success of primary closure and continuous irrigation of the perineal wound in achieving wound healing after proctectomy... We conclude that primary closure with irrigation of the perineal wound is safe and provides satisfactory healing in most patients.[207]

Joseph Pujol (hero extraordinary of French scatology) in his shows demonstrated many types of farts i.e. young girl, mother-in-law, bride. He could even extinguish a candle, 30 centimeters away through his farting.[7]

Irrigation of wounds to remove bacteria and foreign material is an essential of wound management along with debridement. The effectiveness of saline lavage by high pressure (50 psi) pulsatile jet irrigation has been compared with conventional gravity flow and bulb syringe procedures... Irrigation diminished bacterial counts in all wounds, but only pulsatile jet irrigation brought about significant reduction of bacteria in each type of wound... clean contaminated wounds were infected at three days but not at seven days after lavage, while traumatized wounds remained infected at ten days except for those initially irrigated by pulsatile jet. Thus, pulsatile jet irrigation removed bacterial from experimental wounds more efficiently than conventional procedures.[106]

Another part of our anatomy also gives us more information on water jets cleaning injured or infected tissue. The skin in our mouths is not dissimilar to skin in our colon. Both are in difficult healing situations, being constantly washed with food and bacteria. Since the 1960s water picks (basically a bidet in this function) have been used to heal wounds, both gingivitis and periodontal, in your mouth. It seems to me that the following studies indicate the potential for bidets in wound cleaning and repair. They promote a water pick jet whose pressure varies from 50-90 psi, much higher pressure than the pulsed lavage described above for post-surgical cleaning at 15-50 psi.

Debridement of necrotic tissue is essential for healing open or infected wounds. The Water Pik is a therapeutic device that assists in the removal of necrotic tissue. The Water Pik is inexpensive, easily available, and may be used with few contraindications.[96]

Evaluation of the safety of a water flossier on gingival and epithelial tissue at different pressure settings. From this, the researchers concluded that up to 90 psi was acceptable on undamaged oral tissue while 50 to 70 psi was recommended for inflamed or ulcerated tissue. Selting et al found that efficacy was similar between medium and high pressure settings, but at lower settings it was 50% less efficient... The primary physical action from a dental water jet has been shown to occur subgingivally... Other researchers have also found bacterial reductions showing the dental water jet disrupted spirochetes up to 6 mm... The specimens were microscopically evaluated and the irrigated tissue was found to have less inflammation, better connective tissue organization and greater keratin layer thickness in irrigated tissue compared to non–irrigated areas.[209]

Why Not a Sitz Bath?

A typical sitz bath or a traditional stand-alone bidet (with standing water) is much less hygienic than free-flowing tap water. Though such sitz baths are often prescribed as part of the healing process, if the water used for wound care is not clean, a new or worsening infection may occur. Sitz baths (or bidets) with circulating, ever fresh water do not engender this possibility. Consider your alternative; toilet paper can introduce bacteria, cause irritation, or leave a residue.

Conclusions: This study shows that sitz bath does not offer pain relief, wound healing or reduction in consumption of analgesics and thus there is no evidence to prescribe sitz bath in the post-haemorrhoidectomy period.[214]

[Sitz bath: where is the evidence?] Thirty-six articles were found which highlighted the physiology, benefits, risks, complications, and techniques of sitz bath. Most of the studies were published in gynecologic or nursing journals... Five articles reported complications of sitz bath, including dissemination of herpes, maternal-neonatal Streptococcus outbreak, and skin burns. CONCLUSION: A review of the literature demonstrated a lack of scientific data to support the use of sitz bath in the treatment of anorectal disorders.[213]

A sitz bath with circulating water still lacks the other features that make bidets attractive. Read more about sitz baths in **Traditional Bidets and Sitz Baths in Health.**

However, the [bidet] group reported significantly greater convenience (p < 0.05) and higher overall satisfaction (p < 0.05) compared with the sitz bath group. At the end of the 4-week postoperative follow-up period, 90% of patients in the [bidet] group and 93% of patients in the sitz bath group showed complete wound healing. There were no significant differences in postoperative complications between groups... The results demonstrated that the water spray method could provide a safe and reliable alternative to the sitz bath for post-hemorrhoidectomy care. Furthermore, the water spray method could be used instead of the sitz bath as a more convenient and satisfactory form of treatment.[42]

Patients undergoing chemotherapy and radiation therapy for cancer have a suppressed immune system. They frequently experience long bouts with severe diarrhea, which often leads to skin breakdown and possibly major infections. In addition to relieving the pain and discomfort associated with tender tissues, the Hygenique Sitz Bath can play a major role in reducing life-threatening infections [Oncology Supervisor].[19]

We primarily use the Hygenique Sitz Bath system for rectal surgeries and some GYN procedures, and it has been very effective preventing infections with both. Nurse Manager.[19]

It is all in how you use your bidet

Anal hygiene after defecation was most commonly done with dry toilet-paper (55%). A change in anal hygiene after defecation relieves symptoms: By changing from water to moist toilet paper in 9%, from dry toilet paper to moist toilet paper in 30%, from moist toilet paper to water in 32%, an from dry toilet paper to water in 60%. These results confirm known facts regarding the influences of conserving agents and printing materials in dry (often recycled) and moist toilet papers on the skin. These side-effects to be even more pronounced in the compromised skin and suggest that anal hygiene should be done with water only.[43]

Seventy-nine (230) individuals were using the warm-water washing toilet seat. There was no significant difference in age between the usage group and the non-use group. The purposes of use after defection, for defecation induction, and after urination were 90.4, 41.3, and 40.4%, respectively. Regarding the kinds of washing, a strong tendency for the use of the anal washing function to induce defection and after defection was observed, whereas a tendency was observed for the use of the bidet function after urination and for washing the vagina.[20]

It is well known that in antiquity medicine often resorted to the use of enemas and rectoclysis to "free" the body of the "humors" and "poisons" believed to originate in the intestine and to cause diseases in many other organs. Indeed, an Egyptian papyrus dating back to the XVI century B.C. provides evidence of the belief that toxic substances produced by poorly digested foods could pass through the intestinal lumen and into the blood stream causing disorders even in distant organs. In summary, the regular use of colon cleaning techniques could, in individuals with serious intestinal motility problems, be an effective part of the stability of intestinal microbiota.[289]

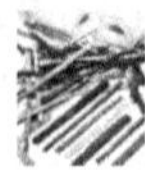

Doctors Are Late Catching Up

A recent e-mail from a reader wondering whether bidets make good sense for older people caught my attention, though – primarily because it came from Dr. Mary Tinetti, chief of geriatrics at Yale Medical School. By chance, she'd heard from several colleagues and family members who were praising bidets as a safer and more effective way for the elderly to clean themselves. "It made me think, 'Why isn't this more broadly recognized?' " she told me in an interview... "Bathrooms are dangerous places for people with poor mobility and balance — there are all those hard, wet surfaces. If older adults can take fewer showers and baths, using the bidet to wash their lower bodies and a washcloth and soap for their upper bodies, they might reduce the risk of falling, Dr. Tinetti said... "As people get older and frailer, it's harder for them to do good personal hygiene, particularly if they have arthritis," Dr. Tinetti said. "They can't maneuver around" to wipe or wash themselves effectively. In their attempts, they can even fall from the toilet [2012].[257]

"Bidets have health benefits?" (Uttered by a proctologist when I told him about this book).[44]

Ecology of the Bidet

The ecology and efficiency of the bidet is clearest when compared with TP, which will become clear in the second part of this book, but examples abound throughout this book.

Increased Efficiencies of Bidets

Everything you think you know about defecation is wrong. the stone cold truth is that we're dealing with the same piece-of-crap toilet technology that was invented in 1596.[69] From 1880 onwards, however, the emphasis (on flush toilets) has been more on aesthetics to make cisterns and bowls decorative.[7]

"Basically, the huge industry of producing toilet paper could be eliminated through the use of bidets," offers Thomas, who has been testing different toilet-seat mounted units for the past two years. He would like to someday pair a bidet with a composting sawdust toilet for the ultimate green bathroom experience.[20]

Throughout the world, Japan's space-age toilets are about as well-known as Godzilla, sushi and Pokémon. Heated seats, massage functions, pressurized water sprays for rears and lady gardens alike; those toilet seats have everything a visitor to the bathroom could ever dream of, and, for me at least, there are few things in life more pleasing than opening a bathroom door to be greeted by a high-tech toilet springing to life and begging me to sit on it to do my dirty business.[114]

Bidet efficiency has benefited greatly from the evolving technology. As an example, let's look at heated water, available on the more advanced units. At first customers would complain that it took too long to heat the water or that the water temperature would suddenly rise and fall. These deficiencies were overcome by improving the on-demand heater and by providing a temperature control device that employs a sensor.

Models currently on the market have temperature control buttons for the bidet water, deodorizers, heated seats, fans that "break down odorous molecules," digital clocks to tell users how long they have been on the toilet, a control panel that offers a choice of flush strengths, and devices that automatically put the seat down when you are done. When Madonna visited Japan for the first time in 12 years in December 2005 she said she longed for Japan's warm toilet seats.[184]

I totally dig the bidet concept. If you are going to use one, I recommend you go high-tech. One time I was staying in this Japanese owned hotel in NYC and they had DIGITAL BIDETS. It was soooo fucking cool. All you have to do is press a button and BAM! a cool refreshing drink for your ass. It almost felt like the bathroom of the future, today.[12]

According to a 2019 trends study conducted by the National Kitchen and Bath Association, designers consider a toilet with a bidet squirting feature the most important thing to put in a new bathroom today, with more than half of the 500+ designers surveyed saying they install cleansing toilets as opposed to regular ones, for clients. Bidet seats and bidet toilets in the U.S. are currently a $106 million category expected to grow 15 percent annually through 2021.[3]

There are literally hundreds of bidet models available. On a budget and freaked out over the stories of bidet units that are thousands of dollars? There are many fine units under $100. There's no breaking the bank when it comes to providing people with a cleaner butt. However, the power is in your hands!

 From the Urban Dictionary: Bidet: An automatic ass cleaner using water at a water temperature and power of your choice. Can be installed as a completely different commode or in the same toilet seat itself. The evolution from using standard toilet paper and digging into your arse hole to remove that brown excrement. "If you're still using toilet paper you're living in the 19th century and beyond. Wake up you bastards and get a bidet. NO HANDS needed to dig into your ass. When your done hosing your ass down, just PAT dry with a single square of TP".[45]

Ecological Savings

When considering everyday habits and practices with a harmful environmental impact, toilet paper use would not be the first activity to come to mind. The use of toilet paper in Western countries is a very common habit and in most sanitation environments the only option of cleaning after using the toilet.[66]

Bidets are usually a simple add-on to people's existing municipal water and sewage plumbing, or to rural septic systems. Bidets counteract many of the worst effects of the TP/flush toilet combination. Admittedly much of the profound ecology of bidets comes from ameliorating the extreme anti-ecology of TP/flush toilet use enumerated in a following chapters on TP vs. Our Environment.

The Centers for Disease Control and Prevention estimates 80 percent of all infections are transmitted by hands. Frequent hand washing can help curb the spread of flu and other conditions, which costs the nation more than $83.3 billion each year in lost productivity and medical bills.[272]

It is important to note that bidets use very little water; much much less net use of water (less pollution) than flushing with TP! Many bidets use no toilet paper at all (and at worst much less), a huge ecologic saving. Using a modern bidet with self-cleaning features is much cleaner and health-preserving than using a standard toilet. Bidets can minimize your need for baths or showers, while keeping you cleaner overall.

Sabrina Foulke, architectural designer at Point One Architects + Planners in Old Lyme, Conn, ""[Toto Washlets are] basically the only toilets we recommend at this point," Foulke says. "They have a toilet seat that's also a bidet. They've also addressed the flushing mechanism, which nobody had redesigned in 100 years. The toilet functions very well, it uses less water, and you get the option of the seat that can function as a bidet; it's a heated toilet seat—it'll do everything. It's scary. I actually have a friend who has one, and the heated part is quite nice".[254]

A new type of a stationary robotic toilet is outlined and the concept of the smart interaction between user and envisaged robotic toilet is described. Main functionality are height and tilt adjustment, support of sitting down and standing up, speech interaction, automatic recognition of the user and corresponding preferred settings of the toilet and automatic inference of potential emergency situations. The interaction is challenging due to the very different needs of the target group, the physical contact to the robotic system (actually the user is sitting on the robot) and the taboo area of toileting.[229]

If you press the button after defecation, a toothbrush shaped squirt gun appears from the back of the bowl and begins shooting a stream of warm water onto the anus. Some women may also press the "bidet" button to wash the external genitalia. The pressure of the water stream is adjustable from strong to weak. Finally, you press the button that starts the blow-dryer and wipe off the remaining water with toilet paper.[203]

Kyoji Asada is one of the top toilet designers for Toto. He takes great pride in his job, working 50 to 60 hour work weeks to come up with new innovation and making the rounds of existing toilets to see how they are holding up. Asada told the Washington Post, "Maybe we can't build the perfect toilet. But we can build the toilet that no one has yet imagined. That is our mission".[184]

One happy American owner of a Washlet told U.S. News and World Report, "I shouldn't say this, but sitting on that toilet is actually one of my favorite things of the day now." Other satisfied Washlet owners include Madonna, Brad Pitt, Will Smith, Demi Moore, Bryant Gumpbel and Howie Mandel. Whoopi Goldberg bought six of them for her New Jersey home. She told Barron's, "I'm hooked and I'm spreading the word to my friends." Among the things she adores about them are the heated seats.[184]

David Clancy of DS Construct Inc. in Deerfield Beach, Fla., has installed about a dozen bidet-type seats. He prefers the Toto Washlet. "Maybe 25 percent of my clients will put in a Washlet," he says. "It's not something I push. They aren't cheap." Still, his high-end bathroom projects typically include them. "In the $50,000 range, everybody's getting them," he says. "They'll have a Washlet and a TV in there somewhere. (2009)".[208]

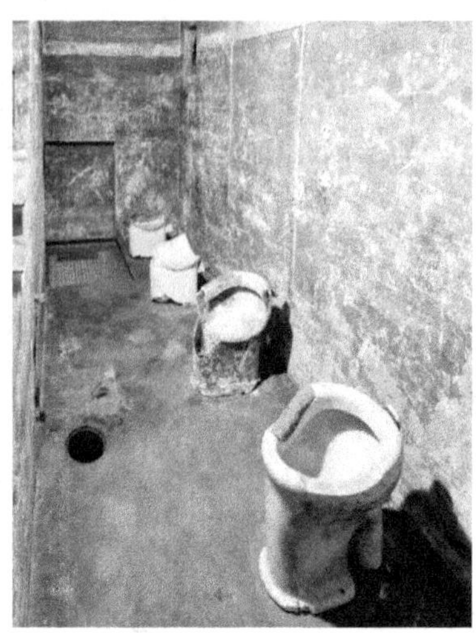

Cleaning With a Bidet

Every bidet will use water to wash your perianal region quite clean. This washing can be completely automatic or can demand significant user involvement depending on the type of bidet you choose. Both approaches have their appeal, and many people opt to have the use of both.

All bidets that are fixed in place generally only require you to turn on a faucet or push a button. With the classic bidet you sit in a bowl flooded with water like a small bathtub and soak yourself clean. With the French bidet and Shower Toilet you have a relatively fixed spray that you adjust to. You usually set up a toilet seat bidet (TSB) once for the optimum spray(s) for your derriere, and it generally repeats this forevermore.

Handheld and traveler's portable bidets offer a maximum of freedom and flexibility but also demand high involvement in the washing process. The potential for unsavory messes is always there for the careless user.

When it comes to drying, the best (and most expensive) shower toilets and TSBs gently and automatically air dry your bottom. For the rest of the bidets, the choice of drying method is made easier because your bottom is at least completely clean. The last part of this section concerns drying methods other than air dry.

"Definitely used for the bootyhole. I've been all around the world and there are all sorts of ass-spraying mechanisms."- Brad W., America[274]

I remember when I first went to Europe and I was like, "what the hell is that thing in the bathroom!"[299]

Traditional Floor Models

Flooded Bowl, French Bidet

How did I get into this? Being an uncouth phone man...the first bidet I ever saw was at the Ritz Carlton Hotel in Chicago where I was fixing wall phones in the bathrooms (the steam would kill the dials). The security guard who was with me had to tell me what these things were. The bidets in the big buck suites were stupid! It's a big porcelain bowl. You turn on the faucets to adjust the temperature, and the water sprays straight up - soaking any clothes you might be wearing!... With the electronic IntiMist, you can wear a suit or dress - it's the same as using a regular toilet! [81]

The original bidets have a vertical spray that comes from the bottom of the bowl. If the bowl was stoppered to accumulate water to soak in, the spray was directly affected. Modern units are often equipped with a horizontal spray that washes you from your genitals back (if you face the wall as traditionally done). This spray is much less precise than shower toilets or TSBs, and generally you must disrobe to use it. I suppose the advantage is that you get a warm wash without a lot of external piping, nor is an electrical outlet necessary. Virtually maintenance free.

Typical Directions for Using Traditional French Bidets

(1) After using the toilet and wiping with toilet paper, you then move over to your bidet. (2) Sit on your bidet, legs astride like on a horse, facing the taps (faucet). (3) While sitting, you simply turn on the water. When the temperature is to your liking, you increase the pressure to direct a stream or spray of water towards those spots in need of cleansing. (4) Cleanse anus and/or genitals. Pat skin dry with toilet paper or towel.

Some models are designed with seats, and the user sits on the bidet the same way they would on a toilet. Controls for any of these models can be at the side or towards the front of the unit.

Greg did the one thing anyone who's installed even one bidet in their history should know to not do. He faced the toilet and said, "So, you turn this knob here to start the water, see?" And with that, the bidet sprayed him, full blast, right in the face. In his open mouth. Water ran down his chin and into his denim shirt. It took him a full two-mississippi to turn the dial to "off." I didn't dare laugh because I felt bad for him. He just got sprayed in the face with hot toilet water. To be fair to Greg, it was fresh water from the tap, the same we drink from, but still. I'd love to say that it didn't happen a second time two minutes later, but it totally did. I was examining the connections, making sure nothing was leaking behind the toilet. I put my hand where I thought the water would hit, to block it from shooting out of the toilet. I turned on the bidet and the stream shot past my hand and directly onto Greg. He was standing in the same spot. He had his mouth closed this time, so it only further soaked his face and shirt. "Sorry," I said to Greg. He shrugged.[90]

I Cleaned My Ass With A Bidet And This Is What Happened: Not that I needed to, because girls don't poop or anything - BuzzFeed Staff

1. Do NOT immediately turn the bidet on full blast. You will not be ready. That is varsity bidet use, and you must work your way up to it.

2. Close your legs. Trust me on this. If your legs aren't closed, the water will find that open space, shoot through it, and splash the opposite wall. I'm a feminist, but still, my advice to you is: close your legs. Sorry.

3. You might have to wiggle. Especially your first time. The water will probably hit the correct general area, but it might not be a blowing-up-the-Death-Star-type shot on your first try.

Yes, you sASSy bitch, it's a bi-DO. Sure, I would love to try one with warm water, but I also know that would require more installation prowess than I currently possess. So I'll wait. I will say, however, that if you are an infrequent wearer of lipstick, it might not be worth it. You probably don't use much toilet paper anyway. But, if you have sensitive skin, hemorrhoids, or a child, you could definitely benefit from a bidet. Also, if you enjoy the feeling of water being sprayed up your butthole, you should get one. Oh fuck, I said butthole.[111]

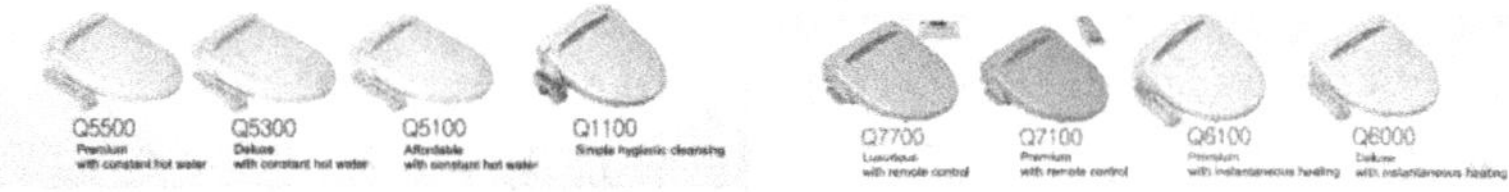

TSBs (Toilet Seat Bidets)

Inexpensive Cold Water TSBs

TSB units can be primitive and cheap, with a single fixed spray that may be adjustable. These days even cheap TSBs have a cleaning jet that the water pressure extends to do the cleaning, and then retracts when the valve is shut off. Most cheap TSBs recommend that you keep the water valve shut off when not in use, in case of water valve leaks/floods.

These units automatically spray to the same spot every time, which may not be your spot, so you may have to adjust your body to benefit best from this spray. The question for any given model should be how effective the spray can be.

Inexpensive TSB bidets usually offer only cold water, which is adequate for cleaning, and has adherents who believe it is the most healthy way to wash. More expensive units offer warm/hot water for additional cleaning power and creature comfort.

I've had mine for five years now. Same brand. It is cheaply made of plastic, but I've had no issues with it. I put another one of my second bathroom. No issues either. Would buy again... My mom's basic Toto model is going on 20 years. My grandma had one that was much older than that... I have the cold water only version of this and it has worked great. Wish there was hot water plumbed near the toilet though as the cold water can be a bit shocking at times.[246]

We got it in July of this year, paid ~$60 for it. It is a very simple one. I liked it because it looks almost exactly like a regular toilet seat. It's fine if you don't mind the lack of temperature control; which I was worried would be a big deal, and turns out so far it has not been an issue, we'll see after this winter if that holds true. No complaints about this unit; it does exactly what it is supposed to do. It's likely that we will spring for a more expensive & fancier one some day, maybe one with a warm-air dryer; but this one gets the job done. The seat I posted above is great so far, but due to the real consequences of water moving through small orifices, this thing, like everything else will eventually get clogged. I did not opt for installing the filters because by my calculation, the filters are more expensive than our bidet-seat-washlet.[246]

Typical Directions for Using Inexpensive TSBs

After defecating, (1) swing the cleansing jet into place, other wise the cleaning jet should automatically project out with water pressure, (2) sit on the toilet seat, (3) turn on the water supply slowly and adjust the temperature if that is an option, (4) otherwise press the wash button, the start button, or open the valve enough to wash, (5) adjust your body for maximum cleaning, (6) turn off the water or press the stop button when finished, (7) wipe dry [I dry with a wash cloth that hardly ever gets soiled], (8) swing the cleansing jet back under the toilet seat if that is needed. Shut off the water supply to the bidet.

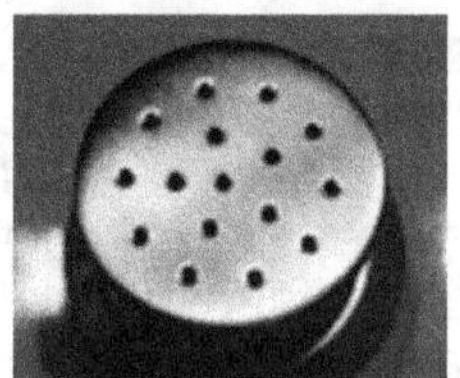

High End TSBs (Washlet)

The higher-end TSB bidets and shower toilets often allow you to select between two (or more) different sprays that come from different directions. For example, you could set up a more concentrated spray to wash away feces first, and then a softer, wider spray from the other direction for cleaning the genitals. This cleaning power can be augmented by a spray that may oscillate, pulse, move back and forth, or use air bubbles. This of course necessitates that you program this unit to fit your particular washing needs, but once done it will repeat endlessly.

Many Westerners are baffled by the complicated array of buttons on a Japanese toilet. Describing an experience that he said was the one of the most embarrassing in his life, an American diplomat told the Washington Post he tried to flush the toilet at the dinner party of a Japanese host, but hit the flushing-noise-maker, the blow-dryer and then the bidet button and "watched helplessly as a little plastic arm, sort of squirt gun shaped like a toothbrush, appeared from the back of the bowl and began squirting a stream of warm water across the room and onto the mirror." He had to spend about ten minutes mopping up the water before rejoining the party. [Source: Mary Jordan and Kevin Sullivan, Washington Post].[184]

Typical Directions for Using A High-end TSB

After you have initially set up the spray wand to wash your derriere precisely how you want it washed, all you have to do is press a button and washing, drying, and deodorization all take place automatically. Subsequently pull up your underwear, completely clean and dry. If you are old, some units will help you to your feet.

Handheld and Portable Bidets

Why would anyone use a handheld bidet when such effortless, automatic bidets are available? One factor is price, balancing a $20 handheld device against a $90+ basic TSB, or a $600+ top-of-the-line bidet. The handheld units are not very visible and take up little space. The big reason for me (and probably most handheld users) is the potential precision and accuracy of my cleaning experience, which puts responsibility on me every time. Properly used they can also help induce defecation. More on this in the **Appendix**.

I just purchased a 2nd [handheld bidet] for other bathroom (yes it's that good). -- It's a shame I waited so long to get one of these. Installed in about 10 minutes, no leaks, works great and feels like quality. The naivety of thinking wet wipes were the cleanest option available. This item is highly convenient and I regret not knowing about it until now. You know, Americans just assumed a bidet was a separate porcelain device; had no idea this affordable hand held existed... This item definitely impresses me and is one of the best purchases I've ever made.[247]

THIS IS THE FIRST PRODUCT REVIEW I HAVE EVER LEFT AFTER MORE THAN A THOUSAND AMAZON PURCHASES. IT IS AMAZING!!! IT MORE THAN LIVES UP TO EVERY CLAIM BY THE MANUFACTURER. I HAVE TWO TOTO WASHLETS (TOILET SEAT BIDETS) AT $1500 EACH AND THIS HANDHELD DOES A SIGNIFICANTLY AND CONSISTENTLY BETTER JOB IN 10 SECONDS THAN MY WASHLETS DO IN 60 SECONDS. EASY TO CONTROL WITH MORE THAN ENOUGH PRESSURE.[247]

Handheld units offer you perhaps better (or worse) washing than most fixed units. Much better when a practiced hand can apply the spray with surgical accuracy, a watery smelly disaster if carelessly used. Handheld units can be much worse at washing when the beginner's hand can make a significant, disgusting mess by blasting feces all over the toilet area. The key to using a handheld unit cleanly is sensitivity and accuracy. I would also recommend that you check the toilet lid top and bottom every time you use a handheld bidet, especially when you first start using a handheld bidet. If I do not check, then every once and awhile I get this shocked disgust from my wife in the bathroom. Best not to go there.

Handheld Spray Technique

Learning To Shoot: This is not silly nor flippant, you have to learn to shoot a handheld spray. The goal is always to keep the spray upward and pointed over and towards your anus, and away from your genetilia. I reach through my legs all the way under to my anus and squirt slightly backwards from there. For those of you who cannot achieve this contortion, there are handheld bidets with an extension that points everything correctly from your legs to your anus.

Wash Front to Back: At first I tried washing back to front. I would lean forward and hold the sprayer at my back, and start spraying from the top of my buttocks' crack forward. My body at this point is in as close to an ideal crouch position as is possible on a toilet.[8]

This worked pretty well, kept any over-spray in front of me and very visible, but I had to abandon that approach. No matter how careful I was, some of the spray was depositing some fecal material on my genitals, and I started to have some skin problems. Soon after I stopped doing this, the skin problems stopped.

For over 16 years now I have been spraying from the front to the back, and I am completely satisfied with the results. When I changed my spraying technique, I replaced the round toilet seat with a u-shaped one that has a gap in the front. This opening makes it much easier to reach through my legs and past my genitals to wash my anal region. You have to learn how the contours of your derriere both reflect and concentrate the water spray. Spraying gently up the anal fissure from over the anus but angled away from my genitals, minimizes destructive side-sprays and removes the fecal matter safely. Controlling the spray pressure is crucial, especially with muni systems. With experience you can then feel more confident in spraying the area a little closer and a bit more force to the cleaning.

The first goal is to remove as much of the fecal remains as possible, at as low a pressure as possible, minimizing the chance of splatter and creating a mess. Experiment with the lowest water pressure that provides effective cleaning.

Using a handheld bidet demands that you be careful and accurate. It takes very little misdirection of the sprayer to leave a messy puddle on the floor next to the toilet/bidet. Any over-spraying is directed towards the back and is thus easy to overlook. Again, begin spraying gently, removing most of the fecal matter with the least amount of kinetic energy, offering the least opportunity to create a mess. The most dangerous times for a mess are when you have diarrhea.

People have died from pooping too hard. It caused their blood pressure to rise enough to shake loose a blood clot or burst an aneurysm.[297]

I would also recommend pulling up your shirt or blouse in the back. While the spray usually stays within the bowl, a shirt/blouse hanging down can get wet, since some can drape down close to (or past) the anal fissure. It is easy enough to measure how low any given garment goes, but to be safe I just hitch it up above my waist.

If Your Goal is to Induce Defecation

Using a bidet to induce defecation is not recommended, particularly if you have any conditions in your perianal area that might be made worse by attempting this. It is strongly recommended that you consult your health practitioner before considering this. Nevertheless, if your goal is to help induce difficult or constipated defecation refer to the **Appendix.**

When my daughter was three to five years old, she and her friend regularly used the bidet as a Barbie swimming pool. Unfortunately one day she put her Rachel doll (S Club 7) into the bidet to swim. Normally when Rachel's arms were lifted, she sang "Reach for the sky". Sadly she never sang again. Copenhagen, Denmark.[23]

Ensuring Cleanliness with your Handheld Bidet

If you intend to try a handheld device right away, there are ways to minimize your chances of creating a mess. Almost all of the errant spray that spills out of the toilet comes through the space between the toilet seat and the toilet bowl. I do not know why this space is actually there, but it is a major problem for the beginner. I never tried this, but you could try attaching a shield to the toilet seat that extends past this gap and a little into the toilet bowl.

Toilet seats are cheap, and it would be worth it to purchase a cheap one to modify as your "training wheels." You could simply remove the spacers on the toilet seat that cause this gap, though you will probably have to temporarily remove or replace the toilet seat hinge as well. You can then restore your usual toilet seat when accuracy is no longer an issue.

For family and domestic bliss, be sure to always check under the toilet seat, between the toilet tank and the toilet body, and the sprayer itself. Clean up as needed - once you are fully experienced, messes are infrequent, but it should not be others who discover this or clean it up.

If money is not an issue, it might be worthwhile to purchase an inexpensive TSB (toilet seat bidet) just to get used to the process of washing, before you attempt to try the wild freedom of the handheld device. Contrariwise, it might be handy to have a handheld unit even if you have a TSB, or even if you own a classic or French bidet.

Drying Techniques

So you are clean but your butt is wet. There are times where I have known that my bottom is clean and simply pulled up my underwear and pants and allowed my body heat to slowly dry things out. Frankly I find that pretty uncomfortable. Realistically you have three options: have a bidet that air dries, employ a reusable cloth or towel, or use toilet paper/towel to pat yourself dry. I personally use a dry washcloth and rotate it with every wash, although usually it is not obviously soiled at laundry time.

In the decade 2007-17, RCF consumption by tissue producers has grown by 3 million tons, while market pulp for tissue has grown by 8 million tons. Meanwhile non-wood fibres have held onto their niche purposes, but their consumption is apparently gradually eroding over time.[250]

Air Dry

The more expensive TSBs and the Shower Toilet offer a warm air drier for completely hands-off operation, which insures optimal personal hygiene. They generally heat the air that is drying you. If I ever break down and buy a real bidet, this would be a necessary feature to get my wife involved.

The bidet is the best thing since sliced bread. First saw one in England- had no clue what it was - and thought it was weird and a little intimidating. Then I tried it, and was an instant convert. Loved it so much, in fact, that we had one installed in our new master suite, and now my husband uses it, too. An interesting side note- I used to get the occasional bladder infection, but haven't had a single one since I started using the bidet.[12]

Neil A. Martin of Barron's called the Toto $5,000 Neorest 550---the Maserati of plumbing. "As you approach the lid rises in greeting. The seat heats up. A catalytic converter snaps to attention ready to absorb the faintest of unfortunate odors, Then you pick the sound effects---anything from Mozart to simulated toilet flushing to the crash of ocean waves. Folks in the living room may wonder what's going on in there-but at least they won't hear something worse. Toward the end a robotic bidet arm swings into action. We'll skip the details except to say that its completes its duties with a warm-air dryer. As you take your leave, the lid closes and Neorest automatically flushes".[184]

Rag or Towel

My personal solution is to use a heavy dark colored wash cloth to dry my behind and then replace it every washday. A second wash cloth is then put into use, effectively rotating the two between clothes' washings. You might very well need at least a third washcloth while learning this method. Once you are experienced with your bidet, these cloths are less soiled than underpants. Just about the only time I have serious soilings have been due to diarrhea.

At first, it was surprisingly difficult to know where my anus actually was, in terms of getting it clean. There were times when I thought I was clean, and wasn't, thus soiling the wash cloth. This pretty much only happens now when I have some diarrhea. This is what is called a "feedback loop," where the evidence of my wipe cloth gets me to wash a little longer and better. After the first few months, I learned how to wash properly, and now routinely send a "clean" washcloth through the laundry.

I suppose there still are some germs on this "clean" washcloth, even if it looks perfectly clean. I believe that letting the washcloth dry between uses eliminates any germs once it dries; germs generally cannot survive on a dry washcloth. Desiccation or dryness kills germs.[82] Laundry washing then ensures cleanliness.

Microbes can live on household surfaces for hundreds of years. The good news, however, is that most don't. Some well-known viruses, like HIV, live only a few seconds. Because viruses must invade cells of a living host to reproduce, their life spans outside are generally shorter than that of bacteria, which reproduce on their own. Humidity also makes a difference; no bacteria or virus can live on dry surfaces with a humidity of less than 10 percent. Of course, any sort of nutrients (food particles, skin cells, blood, mucus) retained helps microbes feed and thrive, which is why your kitchen sponge is such a breeding ground for pathogens.[82]

I hang my wash cloth on the pipe that provides the water supply for the toilet tank. It is a good place to hang it because it is out-of-the-way, not particularly noticeable, but not too far back to grab when I need it. Stuffing it lightly into this u-shaped pipe keeps it in place, yet still loose enough to allow it to dry between uses.

If you are anxious about additional hygiene, I suppose you could use a cloth that on one side had some coating or material that made it impermeable to water, or perhaps a hand mitt. Perhaps a thicker cloth would feel more hygienic. The bottom line is that if hygiene is that much of a concern, this may not be the best bidet to use, since other bidets are available that never require you to touch your rear end. The other bidets give you guaranteed hygiene.

Use Toilet Paper or Paper Towels to Dry

See the next section of this book that exposes the slowly evolving disaster that is coming from our use of TP. It would be a great start for our future to cut our use of TP in half (and Kleenex and paper towels and wet wipes and diapers of all sorts as well) or at least switch to good recycled TP.

Keeping Your Bidet Clean

Keeping most bidet units clean is fairly easy. Original and French bidets tend to wash themselves clean, and I suppose need maintenance on the same schedule as your toilet, depending on how you use them. Handheld and travel bidets require little care, depending on the skill and experience of the operator; some prefer a hygienic wipe after each use. Adding a shut-off valve makes a handheld detachable for easier cleaning, and a fail-safe against inevitable leaking. The most primitive TSBs require cleaning because they are constantly exposed. Keeping the underside of the toilet seat clean requires periodic monitoring. Ceramic or metal units (usually stainless steel) are easier to keep clean than plastic units.

The shower toilet and the better TSBs have robust self-cleaning functions. These TSBs often have a removable main unit that has been designed for easy cleaning. These features are designed to make it simple for consumers to care for and clean their TSBs. They probably can be maintained on the same schedule as your toilet.

General Bidet Cleaning and Care

Keeping your bidet clean can be as simple as pie, or it can be fairly complex; you can choose a bidet model that perfectly matches your toileting needs. Stand-alone bidets (Classic and French) are in many ways the easiest to care for, but do not offer the additional benefits that come with toilet-seat bidets (TSB). This section on bidet cleaning and maintenance is in three parts: general care that generally applies to all bidets; care for stand-alone bidets (also includes all-metal bidets), and care for TSBs

About Cleaning Materials

It's pretty sad a SO DEVELOPED COUNTRY as USA keeps those disgusting habits of spreading shit with paper toilet. Bidets are just so necessary as sinks and toilets. I just can't understand why americans don't wash their intimate parts just after pee or pooh. Are Americans porks???[216]

Do not use a dry cloth or toilet paper on plastic parts. Scrubbing pads and powdered cleaners can scratch the surface of almost any bidet. Strong chemicals, such as bleach, acidic or alkaline cleansers, thinner, and benzene could also damage its surface. When in doubt it would be best to check with the manufacturer of your bidet to determine if it safe to use any particular product.

Success with cleaners and procedures is dependent upon such factors as the hardness and temperature of the water, using exact measurements of ingredients, changes in cleaning formulas and the condition of the product being cleaned. Keeping a cleaning cloth and pack of disposable gloves near the bidet can help encourage all those using the bidet to keep it clean.

The number of Americans without indoor plumbing is OVER 1 MILLION. [122]

Wear gloves if you have sensitive skin. Always allow plenty of time to let one cleaning product air out before using another to clean the bathroom. For example, if you clean the toilet with bleach [a no-no, see below], and then clean the mirrors with your favorite window cleaner. It is dangerous to mix cleaning products, especially if you are mixing ammonia and bleach, which creates hydrochloric acid, which can be deadly. Avoid using aerosol products. Do not allow abrasive chemicals and cosmetics (fingernail polish, aftershave and perfume) to come in contact with the toilet seat, as they can damage the finish.[303]

Bleach is a popular cleaning agent, but many bidets are made out of materials that may be damaged by bleach. What makes bleach such an effective cleaner may also damage your bidet's surface. I have noticed several online sources recommend bleach as the main bidet cleaning agent; I do not recommend that you use bleach until you are sure it does not damage your bidet. Generally it is recommended that you do not clean your smart toilet or bidet with bleach.[301]

General Care

Cleaning a bidet is not any more difficult than cleaning a shower or toilet, but the approach is different. Before cleaning, flush the toilet or bidet. Unplug the power plug if that applies. If the power is not unplugged, the unit may short, malfunction, or cause a failure or electric shock.[304]

Always test your cleaning solution on an inconspicuous area before applying to the entire surface for the first time. Wipe down the surface of your bidet with a soft cloth (or a sponge) that has been soaked in water or an all purpose cleaner. Wipe surfaces clean and rinse completely with water immediately after applying cleaner. Rinse and dry any overspray that lands on nearby surfaces. Do not allow any cleaner to soak.[303] Don't forget to clean the front and back of the lid. [TSBs: Be careful not to let water seep inside or leave detergent in the gap between the top unit and bowl unit. May damage plastic parts or cause a malfunction].

If your SWASH seat or bidet toilet attachment starts looking a little worse for the wear, all you need is a sponge and a mild cleaner like Simple Green or Windex. Harsh, abrasive cleaning products like thinner, benzene, acidic chemicals, chloride, or hydrochloric acid detergent could corrode metal parts and discolor or scratch your beautiful bidet.[300]

In December 2006, Matsushita introduced a new self-cleaning toilet, costing between $2,500 and $3,500, that is made from a new glass material and is said to never need cleaning. Toto has developed toilets with a tornado-like flush and cleaning cycle that wipes away all waste from the toilet and offers an extra wide seat for sumo wrestlers.[184]

(Classic bidet) How could you possibly think that sharing a bidet is gross? That's like saying using the sink someone else has used is gross. Not to mention you just got off the toilet someone else -crapped- in. No part of your body even needs to come in contact with the bidet. And the models I've seen in Europe have a horizontal spray that arches over the water and is caught in the bowl, so no worries of recycled rinse water. When you think about it, toilet paper is pretty unsanitary. You wouldn't just wipe off your hands with a paper towel and call them clean.[12]

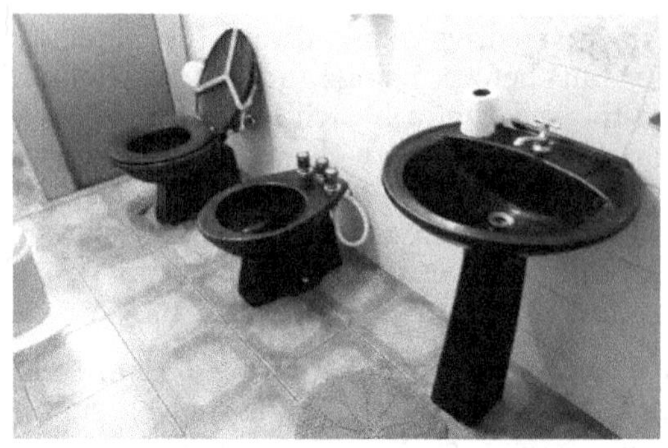

Classic and French Bidets

Classic and French bidets are made from vitreous china, the same as your toilet and sink. These bidets can be cared for in much the same way as your toilet, and can be included in your usual toilet upkeep. Many metal bidets can also be cleaned in this way, avoiding abrasives whenever possible.

Soft abrasive cleaners should only be used when necessary to clean vitreous china products and most metal bidets since strong abrasive cleaners will scratch and dull any surface. Most toilet bowl cleaners are safe to use on vitreous china. Follow label directions and use toilet bowl cleaners on the inside of the bowl only. I do not recommend using in-tank toilet cleaners as they can damage the flush valve or other working parts. Wipe any splashes of any strong cleaner solution if plastic or plated surfaces are part of your bidet.

When using a toilet cleaner to clean the bidet, wash it off within 3 minutes and leave any toilet seat or lid open. Wipe off any cleaner (especially bleach) that remains on the bowl unit.[304]   Your general cleaning should include: Top and bottom of the seat, Rim, Pedestal, Outer bowl, and Tank.

Brushing Technique: Scrub the interior of the toilet or bidet with the toilet brush. Scrub under the entire rim of the toilet or bidet. Gradually spiral the brush down towards the waterline, scrubbing as you go. Once you reach the chute, insert the brush into and out of the chute several times.

Over time hard water deposits may clog toilet rim holes and trapways. To clean, purchase a commercial cleaner that's recommended for the removal of hard water deposits. Follow all instructions on the package. Products to Consider for hard water deposits: Clorox Disinfecting Bathroom Cleaner • Comet Bathroom Cleaner • Fantastik Antibacterial Heavy Duty • Formula 409 Antibacterial All Purpose • Green Works All-Purpose • Lysol Bathroom Cleaner • Soft Scrub Gel with Bleach • Soft Scrub Lemon Cleanser • Tilex Bathroom Cleaner • For rust removal • Super Iron Out Rust Stain Remover • Bar Keepers Friend [303]

Of course, humanity has not always depended on long, silky tree fibers (logged from ancient forests or massive monoculture tree plantations, transported hundreds or thousands of miles, bleached with harsh chemicals, air-dried with high-octane machines, and then shipped thousands more miles (again) for personal cleansing.[117]

Bidet toilet seats (TSBs), handheld bidets, and portable bidets are usually constructed with hard plastics like ABS or polypropylene. These plastics are durable and easy to mold making them ideal for many everyday items like toys, chairs, car parts, and.... bidets. These plastic bidet seats usually have a glossy finish and look great on porcelain toilets. To maintain your bidet's good looks, it is important to avoid cleaning with harsh abrasives or chemicals like alcohol or bleach. These cleaning agents can deteriorate the plastic surface and cause discoloration or cracking. Even worse, damages caused by these harsh chemical cleaners are usually not covered under warranty.[302]

Today's TSB bidets offer many different kinds of products with features, improvements, and options galore. Many of these advances come with more electronics, more moving parts, and unfortunately more concerns about care and maintenance. The nozzle(s) and any filters may need special care. If you follow the manufacturer's recommendations you can expect to have one of these puppies keeping your butt clean for decades.

First of all: wipe down the bidet regularly, at least once a week. Wipe the back surface of the toilet seat and the toilet seat cushions with a soft cloth tightly wrung out with water. (Otherwise adhesion of dirt may result in discoloration.) Alternatively, use vinegar or a mild household detergent squirted onto a damp cleaning cloth. Wipe over the bidet with the cloth and let the bidet air dry. Rinse the cleaning cloth immediately after use with hot water to keep it clean.[301]

Manufacturers of lower end TSB bidets and handheld bidets recommend shutting off your bidet when not in use, because the seal around the valve can fail over time and result in a small flood all over your bathroom floor. High-end bidets do not require this, but many require that you to periodically change the filters on your bidet. Toto in addition has something called a "water filter drain valve".

I strongly recommend actually reading the set-up directions and the user's guide (something I tend to avoid), as well as visiting the manufacturers website. I always recommend first checking the caveats and pitfalls in setting up and operation before buying any bidet. Read purchaser's ratings if available. It is worth the effort to properly install your bidet, first to take advantage of all the features offers, second, proper installation maximizes your comfort with the same personal treatment every time thereafter.

If you have an electrically powered bidet, always unplug the bidet before cleaning it. If your bidet model allows you to easily remove the TSB unit, this will greatly ease your cleaning.

If you really want to return the favor to your Swash and give it the same thorough front-and-back clean it provides you, you can easily remove it from the base of your toilet by pressing the Quick Release button on the side of your Swash and sliding it forward off of the mounting plate. This will allow you to get after those tough-to-reach areas and have your seat looking factory fresh.[300]

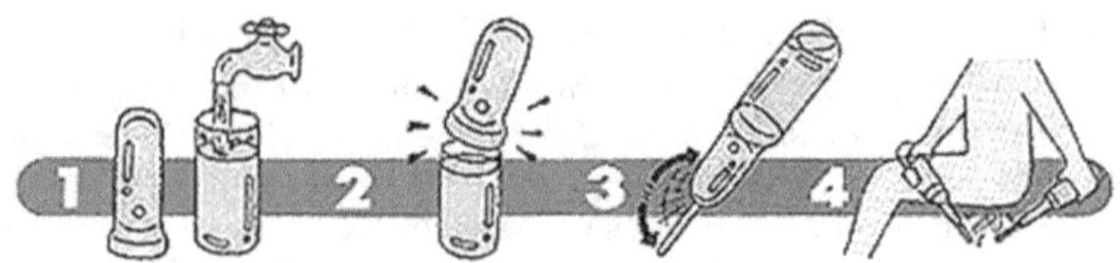

Success with cleaners and procedures is dependent upon such factors as the hardness and temperature of the water, using exact measurements of ingredients, changes in cleaning formulas and the condition of the product being cleaned. The following products are recommended by Kohler for general cleanup: Clorox Disinfecting Bathroom Cleaner • Comet Bathroom Cleaner • Green Works All-Purpose • Green Works Bathroom Cleaner • Tilex Bathroom Cleaner • Windex Original [303]

Cleaning Your Wand/Nozzle(s)

Perhaps the most important and hardworking component of any TSB bidet is the nozzle. This thin, appendage-like probe (or probes) juts out beneath you and does all the dirty work after you're finished with your own. Nozzles range from your everyday fixed plastic sprayers to some of the most advanced, totally customizable, stainless steel tubes ever conceived for personal hygiene. Many advanced bidet seats and luxury bidet seats even feature multiple nozzles with different functions for feminine and posterior washing. A good reading of the user's manual (at least watch the video!) is important with these units.[300]

Since these little dookie pipes are working in such close proximity to your most delicate and, dare we say, coveted areas, it's obviously very important to keep these little water whistles as clean as possible. Use your TSB's self-cleaning nozzle function if you have it. Many bidet nozzles have a self-cleaning feature, making their maintenance very simple. If this feature is used regularly, you may never need to clean it manually.[303]

Those of you interested in an extra DIY level of sterilization for nozzles will find that many advanced bidets make this easy. Bidet models offer different cleaning features, best referenced in your owner's manual. In nearly all cases using a soft cloth or toothbrush with a gentle home cleaning product like dish soap should do the trick. If the nozzle becomes clogged, you could also use a toothpick. Just remember that any toothpick and/or toothbrush used in your bidet's cleaning is dedicated to bidet duty from then on – but you knew that, right?.[300]

Most advanced bidet nozzles have the ability to self-clean. If your prospective bidet doesn't do self-clean automatically, then you should run the nozzle cleaning feature at least once a month, usually by pressing the cleaning button until the nozzle comes forward for cleaning. Then use water mixed with vinegar and a soft toothbrush to clean the nozzle. Soak a badly clogged removable nozzle tip in vinegar to unclog it. If the nozzle operates under low water pressure, it is far more likely to get clogged.

120,000 tons of waste could be saved if each American household used three less rolls a year, plus, it would eliminate $4.1 million in landfill dumping fees. One tree has significant value. Just ONE TREE.[242]

Advanced TSBs can also feature antibacterial nozzles. Cleaning these nozzles is usually simple – often simply pulling them out and giving them a gentle scrub with a soft cloth or toothbrush. For a more thorough cleaning, or for something lodged in the edges, you can usually unscrew the nozzle tip for a thorough detailed clean. Just don't drop it in the toilet![300] If your unit has a second nozzle, press the button again to extend and clean it as well.[301]

Extend the nozzle using the cleaning button and then unplug the unit so that the nozzle doesn't retract while you're still cleaning the nozzle tip. Carefully remove the nozzle tip by gently wiggling or twisting the nozzle. Leave it in vinegar for 2-4 hours, then scrub it gently with a toothbrush to remove all the water deposits. Reattach the nozzle tip and plug the unit back in.[301]

If the nozzle doesn't have a removable tip, extend the nozzle and unplug the unit, then attach a vinegar-filled Ziploc bag to the nozzle with a rubber band or tape, making sure the nozzle tip is completely submerged in the vinegar. Remove the bag after 2-4 hours clean the tip with a toothbrush, and plug the unit back in.[301]

Toto Wand: (Perform monthly, or if you notice dirt) Press the button "Wand Cleaning" The wand extends and water sprays out for cleaning. The wand automatically retracts after about 5 minutes. While extended, wipe with a soft, wet cloth. Do not pull, push or press the wand with excessive force (May cause damage or malfunction). Press the button "Wand Cleaning" again and the wand retracts.[304]

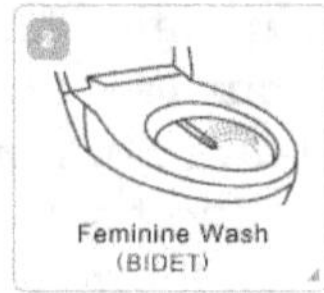

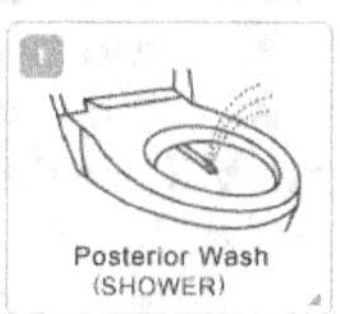

Special Care Checklist

Filters

Most bidet manufacturers recommend a filter (or filters) for the water supply to ensure that any accumulated grit does not clog up the operation of your bidet's nozzle. Grit in my experience can happen anywhere, and also impair the water seal causing a water leak. There might be other service needs explicated in your user's manual.[304]

Many Swash models come fitted with a mesh filter between the plumbing and nozzle. These filters may need cleaning about once a year just so there's no excess particulate matter, grit, or build-up keeping your Swash from running at its full potential. Cleaning these filters is a breeze! All you need to do is unplug the Swash and turn off the water supply, disconnect the Swash from the toilet with the Quick Release button... These filters can be easily scrubbed back to perfection with that same bidet-purposed toothbrush and a little warm water. After you've got the filter looking like new again, place it back inside the water inlet... reconnect the bidet hose, and put the seat back on the toilet. Remember, always consult your owner's manual before doing any cleaning or maintenance to your Swash.[300]

Kohler NOTE: The filter screen should be cleaned once every six months or any time there is a drop in water pressure to the bidet wand.[303]   Service your Toto water filter drain valve every 6 months (Approximately once every 6 months, or if you think the water pressure has weakened).[304]

The following products are recommended by Kohler to clean your filter: Comet Bathroom Cleaner - Green Works All-Purpose - Green Works Bathroom Cleaner - Tilex Bathroom Cleaner - Windex Original - Clorox Disinfecting Bathroom Cleaner [303]

LOL - OMG I can't believe you just post that. I felt like you were waking up the unspeakable - I think that talking about the bidet is almost a blasphemy in the world of bathroom fixtures. (lol) I never saw anybody so irreverent to this innocent piece of ceramic. I had a couple of good laughs - I have to admit ;) This is hysterical! I especially like the bidet as koi pond! Kathy [311]

Removing Tough Stains

Sop up any water inside the bowl with an old towel. Then pour a generous amount of white vinegar inside the bidet bowl. Leave the vinegar in the bowl overnight. Use a cloth dipped in vinegar to remove stains from the edges of the bowl. You can saturate patches of cloth with vinegar and stick them to the stained areas around the edge of the bowl, or any location where the vinegar does not reach directly. Once again, let things sit overnight.[301]

Scrub the bowl with a cleaning cloth to finish removing the stains. Scrub the inside of the bowl with a cloth dipped in vinegar. Then, rinse the bowl with water. Repeat the process if necessary. If your toilet or bidet has rust stains, do not use bleach. Bleach will set the rust stains, not remove them. To remove rust, apply 1/2 cup (64 g) of baking soda to the spot and spray it with white vinegar. Let it react for a minute, then add another cup or two of vinegar. Let the solution sit for 30 minutes, swishing it around a few times with a toilet brush. Scrub the stains until they're gone, then flush it all away.[301]

Do This Every Year

Remove your bidet seat for cleaning at least once a year. You generally do this by pressing the button on the side of the seat or releasing some sort of catch holding it, but your user's manual should tell you how. Once removed clean the bottom of the seat unit with a mild detergent.

Consider replacing the carbon air deodorizer. Unlike aerosols, which block smell with another (more pleasant) odor, carbon air deodorizers filter the air, leaving it free of unwanted odors. To ensure a fresh, clean atmosphere, replace the carbon air deodorizer when it has stopped being effective. Most carbon air deodorizers last a few years and some are designed to last as long as your unit.[301]

Hard water deposits

Over time, hard water deposits may clog toilet rim holes and trapways. If your water resembles this, then an annual unclogging is recommended. To unclog, purchase a commercial cleaner that's recommended for the removal of hard water deposits. Follow all instructions on the package.

The following products are recommended by Kohler for hard water deposits: Clorox Disinfecting Bathroom Cleaner - Comet Bathroom Cleaner - Fantastik Antibacterial Heavy Duty - Formula 409 Antibacterial All Purpose - Green Works All-Purpose - Lysol Bathroom Cleaner - Soft Scrub Gel with Bleach - Soft Scrub Lemon Cleanser - Tilex Bathroom Cleaner   For rust removal: Super Iron Out Rust Stain Remover - Bar Keepers Friend.[303]

Best Way to De-odorize the Bathroom

How do we remove unwanted smells in the bathroom? Most people try to cover up bathroom defecation odors with other smells of one sort or another. People use candles, sprays, and/or some exhaust fan. Candles and sprays don't eliminate the odor, they simply mask it. Some add a nice smelling fragrance to the air in hopes of not smelling the unpleasant one by covering it up.

The better bidets have an internal fan that removes the smelly air produced by your bowel movement before it gets out into the bathroom proper. This air is then run over activated charcoal which very efficiently absorbs the smells and removes them from the air.[187]

Bathroom fans do work and eventaully remove the smell, but they take a long time to work in most cases. Our bathroom has an exhaust fan, but it takes minutes to remove all the smelly air from the bathroom.

Bidet air deodorizers suck the smelly air out of the toilet bowl and push it through a carbon filtration system that adsorbs the offensive smell particles. These bidets are one of the few ways to truly deodorize your bathroom air rather than trying to cover up the odors in your bathroom with other odors.[187,87]

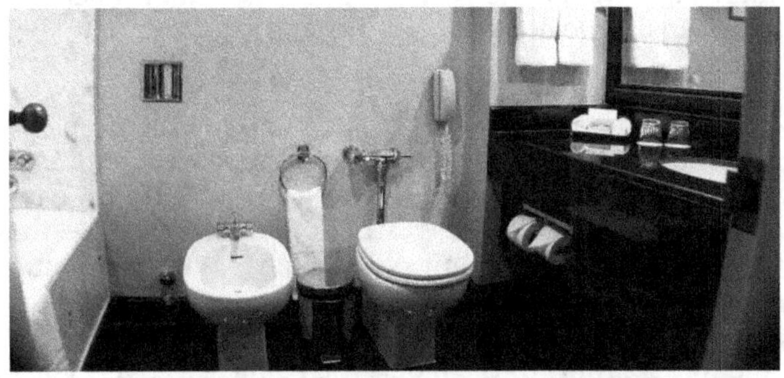

Water and the Bidet

For example, a bidet is used for body washing requires less water than a bathtub or shower. We calculated that a home equipped with a bidet would use, on the average, four gallons a day less than a home with no bidet due to less frequent use of the tub or shower. Likewise, a urinal requires about half the water of a toilet for each flush, so that during a day an average of five gallons might be saved.[91]

It is possible to find electric bidet toilet seats with adjustable pressure options even if you are trying to stay within budget.[188]

Quality of Water

Water is of course essential for any bidet's operation, and the quality of the water you use is of maximum importance. Many of us are fortunate in this country to have drinking-quality water piped into our homes for all our water needs, or supposedly so. Good tap water has been found to not only be quite clean, but also excellent for washing open wounds.[92] Chafed skin (which actually is a very minor wound) thus benefits from rinsing. Research indicates that irrigation, a critical component of wound management, which is commonly performed with sterile normal saline solution, **could be as effective with drinking quality water**.[93]

Tap water samples were collected from different areas within the department and analyzed on two separate occasions for coliforms, S aureus, clostridia, pseudomonas, and beta haemolytic streptococci. RESULTS: Pathogenic bacteria were not isolated from the tap water samples within the A&E department. CONCLUSIONS: Tap water of drinking quality can be used to irrigate open traumatic wounds.[94]

The wounds irrigated with saline had a mean reduction in bacterial count of 54.7%, while the wounds irrigated with tap water had a mean reduction in bacterial count of 80.6%... bacterial decontamination of simple lacerations was not compromised, and was actually improved using tap water irrigation.[95]

The infection rate in wounds cleaned with sterile saline was 10.3% compared with 5.4% in wounds cleaned with tap water... Sterile saline should be replaced by tap water for the cleaning of acute traumatic superficial soft tissue wounds.[93]

Finally, commercially available irrigators such as Water Piks are considered effective wound cleansing devices.[96,97]

Water Pressure

While city water pressures can vary for a number of reasons (variations in elevation, age of system, leaks, and trying to minimize wear and tear), most large cities seem to run their water pressure between 45 and 80 PSI. Our nearest "big city" (Ukiah) recommends installing restriction valves because they run at 90 PSI. This suggests that, if a bidet unit doesn't have a built-in ability to regulate the water pressure, a valve to restrict high water pressure might be a good idea to avoid skin trauma. It might be possible that by partially closing the water valve that controls the water supply to the bidet, you could selectively control the water pressure to the bidet.

The efficiency of wound irrigation is markedly improved by delivering the irrigant to the wound under continuous high pressure. Irrigation of the wound with saline solution delivered at 15 pounds per square inch removed 84.8 per cent of the soil infection potentiating factors from the wound.[105]

I maintain our single-household rural water supply myself. Since we have a small holding tank, the pressure is frequently pumped back up, and runs roughly between 15 and 40 PSI (pounds per square inch). Munis would consider this unacceptably low. This gives me good idea of how variations of relatively low pressures affect my bidet's operation.

A friend is married to a French woman and so understands French bidets. His first experience with a TSB, though, was a cheap unit in a small town in India, where water pressure is chronically low:

"My first experience with a toilet seat incorporated bidet was in, of all places, India, in a fairly cheap hotel. There was a button next to the flush button. I didn't know what it was, so of course I pressed it, and this very small, pretty worthless little stream of water went squirting out of the toilet, across the bathroom, out the bathroom door, and onto the wall opposite the bathroom door of the hotel room. It was impressive, but I couldn't see that it would function very well as a bidet. It definitely needed some work."

"Did you try it?"

"I did try it, but the angle was all wrong because it was shooting upwards so much. Maybe I just needed more practice. I was impressed, though, that they had tried to incorporate it into the hotel bathrooms."

"In most places in India they wash with water, but they just simply have a water tap, and a cup next to the toilet. That has been the age-old system. They usually use their hand in conjunction with the water (to wash their derrieres). It takes a certain amount of pouring skill and a little practice. That's the third world bidet.[104]

A low pressure of 15 PSI is adequate for showers and washing; pre-bidet years we got by with water barely gravity fed by maybe 20 feet of head 100 yards away. And our household top pressure of 40 PSI is more than adequate for all bidet functions, including soft enemas for constipation. I have found that even 40 PSI begins to traumatize my skin after a few minutes of constant spray.

Irrigation of wounds to remove bacteria and foreign material is an essential of wound management... clean contaminated wounds were infected at three days but not at seven days after (irrigation), while traumatized wounds remained infected at ten days except for those initially irrigated by pulsatile jet [irrigated at 50 PSI].[106]

Water Temperature

I wanted a warm water attachment to my bidet so I could blend hot and cold water to suit my needs. For various reasons at the time we built this house, it never happened, and all I have is cold water for my bidet. I haven't really missed the hot water, even in the winter (our water is warmed going through our slab floor, which is also our radiant heating). When I do get cold water it kind of forces the issue. My wife says this is physiologically all wrong, that cold constricts tissue, but the effect on me is like when you go out on a cold day and almost immediately have to go to the bathroom.

If you want warm water, the expense and degree of difficulty depends on the proximity of a hot water source (sink, tub, water heater). Most warm water TSBs have their own electrical water heaters built-in, and thus must have an electrical outlet available.

Cautionary Quote: "Scald burns caused by hot water in the bath are common among the elderly. We present a case of scald burn in the perianal region caused by using the bidet.[107]

The results show a significant effect of the solution's temperature in determining skin irritation. Skin damage was higher in sites treated with warmer temperatures and a highly significant correlation between irritation and temperature was found. In conclusion, the study shows that water temperature during washing has an important effect on the onset of irritant contact dermatitis.[108]

Acute irritant contact dermatitis (ICD) is frequently treated with cool water or saline compresses.[109]

Bidets on the negative side?

One of the underlying assumptions here is that ingestion [of chlorinated drinking water] constitutes the chief route of exposure to the contaminant. Such an assumption disregards other routes of exposure such as skin absorption during bathing or swimming, and inhalation of vapors while showering... skin absorption represents a significant route of exposure. Depending on exposure conditions, it can contribute from 29-91 per cent of the total daily dose, for an average contribution of 64 per cent.... We conclude that skin absorption of contaminants in drinking water has been underestimated and that ingestion may not constitute the sole or even primary route of exposure.[98]

All municipal water these days is at least chlorinated. Chlorinated water used with regularity can pose a health threat. Your skin readily absorbs water and thus some chlorine as well. So long as water contact is relatively brief that is ok. But long exposures, especially warm or hot water, can be a health risk. Using a bidet for an enema puts that chlorinated water in your colon whose function is to absorb excess moisture.[102]

Despite the reported health-related advantages of the use of warm water in bidets, there are health-related disadvantages associated with the use of these toilet seats.... the heat of the toilet seats' warm-water tanks caused heterotrophic bacteria in the source tap water to proliferate inside the nozzle pipes and the warm-water tanks. Escherichia coli was detected on the spray nozzles of about 5% of the toilet seats, indicating that the self-cleaning mechanism of the spray nozzles was largely functioning properly. However, Pseudomonas aeruginosa was detected on about 2% of the toilet seats. P. aeruginosa was found to remain for long durations in biofilms that formed inside warm-water tanks... Infection-prevention measures aimed at P. aeruginosa should receive full consideration when managing warm-water bidet toilet seats in hospitals in order to prevent opportunistic infections in intensive care units, hematology wards, and other hospital locations.[99]

Much research substantiates the medical value of water, irrigation with water, and hydro-massage on the health of the skin, but that presupposes that the water is pure and free of contaminants. My greatest concern would be how much chlorine I would be absorbing using a bidet that draws on municipal water. Out here in the country many of us have our own water source (well or spring) and often use it naturally untreated quite successfully.

Bidets are generally a help in disease prevention; they also can stabilize and help to cure some diseases and conditions. But some modern research out of Japan paints an entirely different picture; without proper maintenance some warm-water bidets can harbor bacteria in their holding tanks.

Bacterial contamination of lavage unit water: Figure 1 gives the mean total bacterial counts from lavage tank water samples taken from 85 households and 28 public facilities. The mean total count from the households was 293±309.1 CFU, while that from the public facilities was 109.5±62.9, showing significantly high lavage tank water bacterial counts in the common household compared to that in the public facilities (P < 0.001). Moreover, P. aeruginosa and E. coli were isolated from the lavage tank water of a number of households.[100]

A toilet's warm-water tank needs frequent inflow of tap water to maintain the concentration of the chlorine disinfectant in the bidet's hot water supply. A residual chlorine concentration cannot be maintained without frequent use. The nozzles of warm-water bidet toilet seats can become contaminated with feces because they are used to wash the area around the anus after defecation. Fecal bacteria have been detected in the bidet's spray water when feces contaminate the nozzle or the region around the hole from which the spray water exits. For example, it is difficult to achieve complete deactivation of P. aeruginosa with the concentration of residual chlorine found in tap water, and there are reports that this bacterium can remain inside biofilms on pipes for long periods.[103]

In recent years, installation of bidet toilets within hospitals in Japan has raised concerns regarding potential for cross-contamination by antimicrobial-resistant bacteria from patients who are hospitalized over an extended period...Of the 292 toilet seats sampled, warm-water nozzles of 254 (86.9%) were found to be contaminated by one or more of the following organisms: Staphylococcus aureus, Streptococcus spp., Enterococcus spp., Enterobacteriaceae and non-Enterobacteriaceae Gram-negative bacteria.[101]

So are bidets cleaner and safer? Millions of people all over the world use bidets that draw on household water and have no obvious problems. Contaminated tap water can be problematical for any cleaning and washing of your body. The research above primarily concerns high-end TSBs that have their own water reservoir, and obviously they need to be cleaned and maintained periodically, or at least used frequently to avoid harboring germs. The latest improvement has been self-flushing tanks and nozzles which hopefully solves this problem.

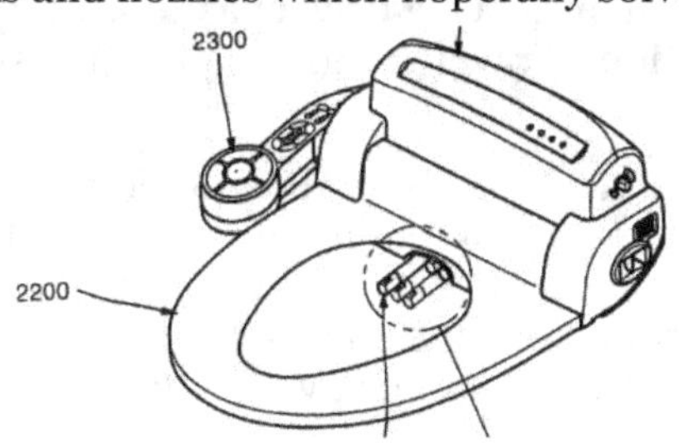

Soap shouldn't be needed with a bidet, and trying to wash your derriere thus would be another whole process. Fifty-two female volunteers washed their hands 24 times a day for 5 days. Five agents were tested: water alone, non-medicated bar soap, a chlorhexidine-containing antiseptic, and two agents containing povidone-iodine (one currently available on the market and one being tested for possible marketing). Some damage to the outer membrane of skin, the stratum corneum, occurred in all groups. Skin damage was determined by the amount of skin shedding, which happens a lot when detergents injure skin. Significantly less such shedding occurred in subjects using water alone... Researchers have found that skin damage occurs during even short periods of frequent handwashing.[110]

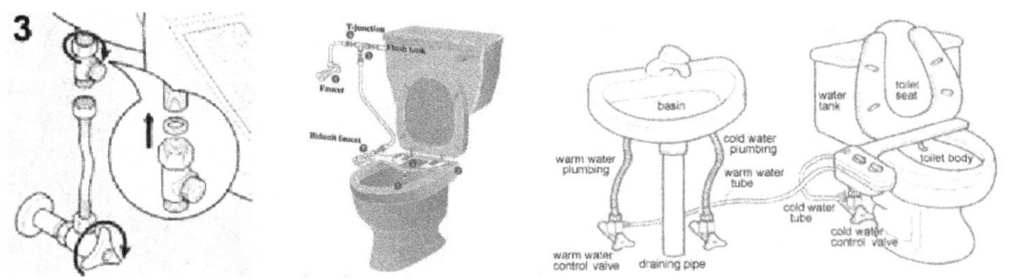

Setting Up The Bidet Unit

Bidets these days are as tough as the 4WD pick-ups that we see bouncing around our back-country roads. Modern materials and manufacturing produce solid, uni-body units with high pressure capabilities, typically rated to 100 PSI or better [but do not attack your bottom with that much pressure - pressure reducer valve recommended]. Most units are made to last a long, long time.

All bidets that I have seen have complete, thorough instructions for assembly. Many manufacturer's websites have videos or animations that make the set-up process crystal clear. In the rare instance that this is not enough, most provide technical help either through the web or over the phone.

The ease of installation depends on the type of bidet. TSBs (toilet seat bidets) and handheld units are very easy to physically install, and come with all the parts necessary to connect up with your toilet's water supply. They usually only need a wrench or pliers (and perhaps a screwdriver) as tools. Many of the better bidets need electricity to function. Travel bidets require no set up, just install the batteries, if needed.

The bidets that are a separate appliance - the Classic bidet, the French bidet, and the Shower Toilet - require major plumbing skills similar to installing a new toilet. Adding a hot water line can be a major project. The following section gives a good general description how the various bidets are installed, with some discussion of what is involved in adding any extra functions.

Installing Classic and French Bidet, Clos O Mat

These are separate fixtures that take up as much space in the bathroom as a toilet. Their advantages are: plenty of room to thoroughly optimize all functions, an utterly sturdy foolproof unit once in place, and a very clean looking installation. All piping and electrical connections come up through the floor, completely hidden. Adding it as a re-model sould be quite expensive.

Installation is significant and time consuming. A building permit is mandatory. Professional installation is expensive. These units are as heavy as a toilet and must be securely mounted to the bathroom floor. Piping fresh water in and draining the wash water out into the sewer (or septic) system requires cutting holes in the floor, plumbing, pipe-fitting, and most likely more permits.

While these are the most expensive bidets, amortization over years of durable, hassle-free use still makes them cost effective. These are a real consideration as part of a new home. Once a house is built, units may have unsightly tubing and wiring that cannot be hidden. Leading manufacturers now produce beautifully designed units - often part of a cohesive, integrated bathroom suite.

These tickle. Hahaha! They definitely give you the "extra clean" feel, but I can't stand the tickling - Walking Tours Rome [69]

It is estimated that roughly 27,000 trees are cut down every single day in order to provide toilet paper for the world, and around 50% of these trees come from virgin forests and old growth specimens that are hundreds of years old or even older. Many of the trees that are used come from primary forests that are sorely needed to help prevent further global warming and increased carbon in the atmosphere. Logging is occurring in forests that are incredibly diverse, and many of these areas contain protected or even endangered species. Toilet paper is filling up landfills in the USA and around the globe at an alarming rate.[87]

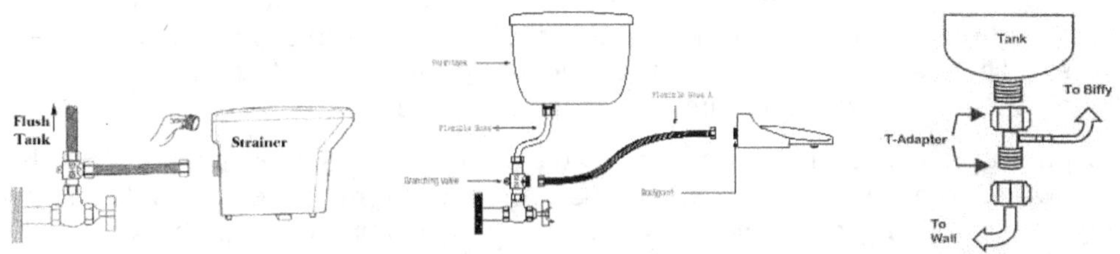

Anything less is uncivilized!... I first tried the bidet seat in a hotel in Japan. To say that something like that was life changing is interesting considering we're talking about a toilet seat but it was. I knew that I absolutely needed to buy one of these when I got back to the states... If you're on the fence about buying one, jump off and buy it. You won't regret it. [1]

The production of virgin wood pulp uses almost twice as much water as producing tissue from recycled materials and generates twice as many hazardous air pollutants.[103]

Installing TSBs, Handheld Bidets

Connecting the bidet water to the toilet water supply always goes like this: (1) Turn-off the valve that supplies water to the toilet, (2) Unscrew the water supply pipe where it connects to the toilet, (3) screw in the supplied T-connector into this same fitting (these are always supplied with the bidet), and (4) the supply pipe is then re-attached to the T- connector. You then have this T- connector that is now sharing the water from the toilet's cold water feed, without interfering with the toilet's regular water supply.

You installed a bidet in a rental unit? It's a bolt-on installation, the bidet replaces the original toilet seat, and the water connection is tied in to the tank connection. When that guy leaves, he can disconnect the bidet in ten minutes and take it away with him. There will be no evidence it was even there. Except the faint intangible feeling that someone with a really squeaky clean bunghole lived there. Dr_Adequate.[84]

Simple bidets that use cold water only are very easy to set up. They have a special connector to tap into your toilet's water feed, and use your home's water pressure to run. The better TSBs heat the cold water with an electric on-demand heater, and have a pump to regulate pressure, thus they need to plug into an electrical outlet.

Some units are designed to be electricity-free and use hot water from your plumbing, which complicates the setup. These usually run one hose from the sink's hot water supply, and another hose from the toilet's cold water supply. This results in a lot of visible piping, but these units tend to run trouble-free and are not subject to electrical blackouts.

That said, leaky valves can occur anywhere along the water's pressurized flow: The junction with the toilet's water supply, the T-fitting that brings water to the bidet, where this fitting attaches to your bidet, as well as the valves in the bidet unit. This is especially dangerous with a handheld bidet. A leak at the wrong time, or over a week's vacation (friends of mine) can really destroy most flooring (and worse). That is why most bidet makers now require the user to turn off the water supply valve when not using their bidet as part of their warranty.

Turning a valve on and off every time you use your bidet is a real pain. If the valve is towards the back of the toilet this would be a major problem for many physically challenged people, this takes away a major bidet benefit. Check the details of the bidet you are buying and see if turning off the water supply is needed under your warranty.

Our water supply comes unfiltered directly from our spring, and so it always contains some grit. This is not a health problem (or hasn't been so far for 38 years), but it can interfere with the efficiency of the water valve, causing it to drip constantly until stopped. Discharging a handheld bidet into the toilet for a few seconds often clears the grit out of the bidet's seal. If that does not work you will probably have to replace the seal, or the unit if it is integral. We have a slab floor so water damage is minimal, so I never turn my bidet water off.

It seems to me that if you have a damageable floor, you could keep the valve on if first of all you had a very good valve, and then either: put in a good filter somewhere in the line to the bidet, or have things situated so that any leak does not end up on the floor. When my bidet leaks my wife puts it in the shower stall.

Handheld units do not necessarily need a water-off valve because they can be stored hanging above the toilet, or stretching into the shower stall, or someplace else that can prevent leak damage.

Read the fine details of the bidet you are going to buy. Look for what the valves are made of. Read any user reviews. How long is the warranty, and what does it cover?

Plumbing Complications for TSBs

There is a possible risk of water becoming contaminated from back siphonage created by the spray fittings. This is an argument for having all bidets installed with a backflow prevention device, if they aren't already part of the unit. Our county requires these. These devices are inexpensive, available at all hardware stores, and simply screw into the water line. Any more complicated procedures should perhaps be taken care of by a professional plumber. Always consult local building codes before installing any plumbing.

If you have copper pipe running to your toilet tank the connection at the toilet tank is probably still a standard fitting. If not, you will have to cut and braze the pipe, and this is surprisingly difficult to do well. A few bidets claim to provide an adaptor for copper pipe, otherwise copper pipe parts are available at any large hardware store. Check the pipe that is the water supply to your toilet. Completely read the directions for the bidet setup you are interested in before buying.

I use these as ice buckets for champagne in hotel rooms and also flower pots. Dr Coustau, Brighton, UK.[23]

There is a standard water cut-off valve for all toilets, and electronic bidets will also have an on/off valve. Nevertheless you might consider installing an additional on-off valve on your bidet water line someplace after the T-fitting. This additional valve is often integral in many bidet units. If you pass on this valve, be sure and leave your handheld unit suspended over the toilet bowl, or in the shower stall in case of leaks.

It would take 51,000 trees per day to replace the number of paper towels that are tossed each day.[242]

This additional valve would be useful for three reasons: (1) You can work on or remove the bidet without turning off the water supply to the toilet (which often involves the whole house's water supply). This is helpful if you need time to repair with the unit; (2) The high water pressures in many cities can be uncomfortable (even dangerous) to use. This valve could lower the water pressure to suit your comfort and needs by partially closing it; and (3) this valve can turn your handheld bidet off to discourage visitors from making a mess when they decide to try out your system when you a not there.

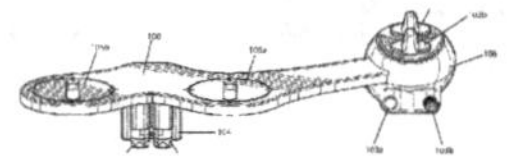

I hope the tiny snippets that are scattered throughout this book express the range of uses that bidets have been put to in people's hands (and butts), and their varied attitudes towards them. I hope that this book expresses to you what people have done with, or experienced through, bidets to give you the best feel for what bidets can be used for, officially and unofficially.

Do (French) bidets have other uses? Yes. They're also used for washing after intercourse and, for us fortunate females, sprucing up during "that time of the month." And, because of their low height, they're great for shaving your legs or washing your feet. (Walk around a historic Italian city in sandals all day, and you'll understand the necessity of that last one)... What do I dry myself with? If you're at a hotel or in your own bathroom, with your personal, hand-sized towel hanging next to the bidet. If you're at a friend's house, with toilet paper. Which brings me to my last point: when in a bathroom in Italy, looking for something to dry your hands or face, don't reach for the towel near the bidet.[89]

Many types of bidet can also be used to clean other parts of the body; they are convenient for cleaning the feet for example. Basically, the Original and French bidets can be used for anything a wash basin is used for. From foot baths, to hand washing clothes, to soaking tennis shoes! The handheld bidets can be used as a spot shower for cleaning. TSBs and true shower closets have limited additional cleaning ability.

A creative person may find uses for his (French) bidet other than ass-rinsing. Crocodile Dundee, for example, washed his boots in one. Last week, my neighbor re-enacted the bombing of Pearl Harbor in his bidet, with tiny model ships. Just last night, I washed my dishes in the bidet.[12]

My handheld bidet is also fine for minor cleaning of the toilet. Angling down the bowl, using maximum water pressure (for me), works best for a clean and tidy touch-up. Minor toilet paper clogs (my wife's) can often be cleared by the jet of my bidet. My bidet also just reaches to the shower stall where it is quite handy for cleaning. Be sure to scrupulously clean yourself after having any contact with the toilet.

Choosing a Bidet

My personal criteria for choosing a bidet would be:

Price (but very negotiable over the right bidet)
Warranty (how long, what it covers). Does it cover leaky valves?
Stability/Longevity of the Manufacturer/Retailer
Multiple Jet Options (the more the merrier)
Heated Seat (implies a reliable source of electricity)
Air Dry (implies a reliable source of electricity)
Self-Cleaning (as much as possible for me)
Helps with Defecation (has controls to do this safely)

Pre-Purchase Considerations

All bidets perform the same basic function of washing your bottom after defecation. The differences are mainly ones of expense, convenience, comfort, or how much mess you can make with it. When in doubt about who to buy from, try to select a reliable long-term marketer of bidets.

Before you purchase your bidet seat, you need to find out what shape your toilet is. A round toilet will be a circle 16.5 to 17.75 inches round while an elongated toilet will have a length of 18 to 19.5 inches.

A bidet seat reservoir comes with a large tank, whose purpose is to heat up water. The issue with reservoirs is that they take up a lot of room and can only heat a set amount of water that's ideal for a one time use. This means that if someone wants to use the bathroom after you, they'll receive a spray of cold water to their posterior. Tankless bidets don't require a tank to heat your water, hence its name "tankless." With those bidets, you can expect a continuous stream of hot water, or at least warm water. If your bathroom doesn't have a lot of room, then the tankless bidet is perfect for you. **Important:** if you have a bidet with a separate water source for heating, and you do not use this bidet frequently, periodically add some disinfectant or change the water.

Having an electrical outlet in the bathroom is a necessity if you are installing a high-end TSB. Do not forget to put in a GFI wall plug if you do.

Proper Feminine Hygiene - Any females who expect to use the bidet in your household will greatly appreciate it if you made sure to purchase a bidet with frontal cleanse. Not all bidets come with this feature, so it's a good idea to keep a lookout for it.[188]

This toilet seat may change the world... I hate to say, but this toilet seat is a game changer. We'll never go back.... Easy to install (if you have power near the water closet) and a pleasure to use for the entire family. This unit includes the seat warmer, which I thought was overkill, but not any more, front and rear water jets, and gentle dryer that makes it totally unnecessary to use messy paper. Prepare for an entirely new experience.[1]

The water seal is an important longevity question to ask your merchant. Do you have to shut the water supply off when not in use? How long do the water seals last? Are they replaceable/repairable? Does this otherwise negate the warranty?

If you have trepidations about spending significant money on a bidet for the first time, consider buying an inexpensive bidet first to try things out. The upfront cost is minimal, and the extra bidet will come in handy at some point.

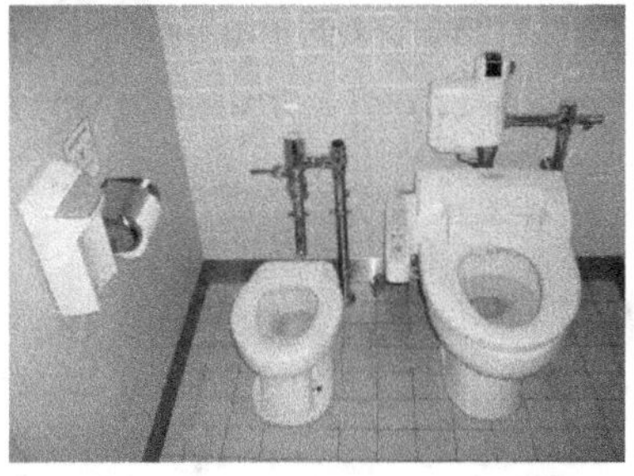

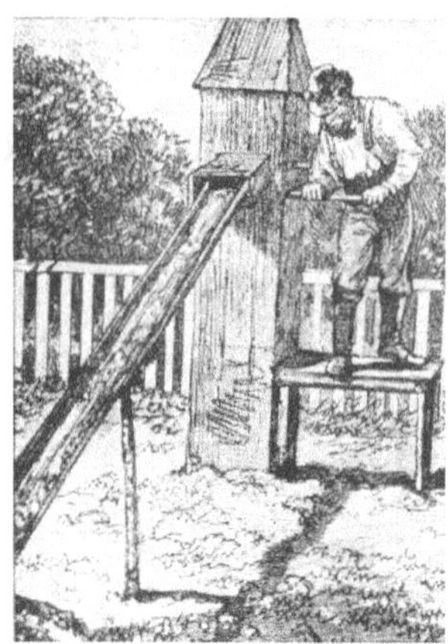 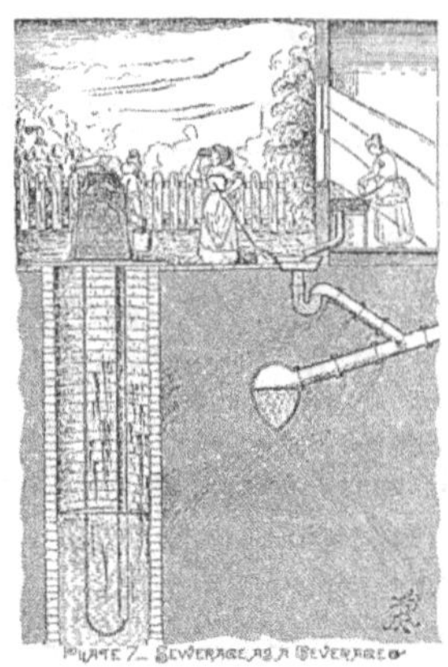

Toilet Paper

TP vs Environment

44% wipe from front to back from behind their backs.
60% look at the paper after they wipe.
42% fold, 33% crumple, 8% do both fold and crumple,
6% wrap it around their hands.
50% say that they have wiped with leaves.
8% have wiped with their hands.
2% have wiped with money![120]

Toilet Paper Fun Facts

The average person is believed to spend three years of their life on the toilet.[122]

If stranded on a desert island with only one "necessity", what would you choose? 49% chose toilet paper as their greatest island necessity (ahead of food!).[69]

What 20th century "convenience" is most taken for granted?
• 69% – TOILET PAPER!
• 42% – zipper
• 38% – frozen foods[119]

If you hang your toilet paper so you can pull it from the bottom, you're deemed to be more intelligent than someone who hangs their toilet paper and pulls it from the top.[53]

People in the USA typically use around 57 squares of toilet paper each day per person.[87]

Americans on average use 23.6 rolls of toilet paper per person every year.[87]

A lifetime supply of toilet paper for one person in the USA requires approximately 384 trees to manufacture.[87,231]

Using a separate piece of cloth to wipe one's nose may have originated during the Roman Empire when people are said to have used linen cloths to wipe their faces and noses.[258]

In the Muslim faith, washing after defecation is concerned with cleanliness and purity of body and soul, and can be applied to both sitting and squatting toilet postures. This comes from the fact that the Islamic culture gives an important role to water in praying, to purify the body and the soul.[125] People from Islamic cultures used their left hand to butt clean with a little water (they are still doing that today). This is why it is offensive to greet someone with your left hand.[53]

It takes 5 gallons of water to flush the average American toilet.[87] A French bidet only requires 1/8 of a gallon of water to clean and flush.[20,87]

The average person will flush their toilet 5 times each day.[87]

The pentagon uses, on average, about 666 rolls of toilet paper every day.[69]

About four billion people don't use toilet paper. About 70% - 75% of the world's population does not use toilet paper. People in some parts of the world do not use toilet paper due to a lack of trees. Some people don't use toilet paper because they can't afford it.[53,87]

Name brand TP is a preference for only 50% of consumers, while 35% reported that they didn't have a preference, and 15% said they didn't know how to answer the question.[231, 242]

Seven percent of Americans steal rolls of toilet paper from hotels or motels.[231]

Stealing toilet paper is a big part of the decision process for commercial enterprises when selecting the kind of dispenser and the type of toilet paper to stock in their restrooms.[53]

It's no secret that Americans have a serious toilet paper habit — the U.S. spent $9.6 billion as a country on TP alone in 2014.[228]

Water is the universal solvent, not paper.[53]

Today bidets can be found in almost every home improvement store in the USA, with prices that are very affordable for typical consumers.[87]

It takes a tree that weighs 1,000 pounds to make 810 rolls of toilet paper on average.[231,242]

Sales in the United States of what the industry calls "luxury" rolls - anything quilted, lotioned, perfumed or ultra-soft, from two- to four-ply - climbed to $1.4 billion in 2014, says the Euromonitor International show. This segment is fastest growing segment of industry.[231]

83 million rolls of toilet paper are produced per day consuming 27,000 trees daily.[242]

The consumer market has many different size rolls. Some rolls only have 200 sheets! Some of the sheets are smaller than the standard industrial size of 4.5" x4.5". I've seen sheets as small as 4'x 3.8". Be careful. Small rolls have to be changed more often and generally do not cost less. Don't get fooled![53]

Traditionally, industrial rolls of toilet paper have 1,000 per roll of one ply and 500 per roll of two ply. Manufacturers also produce jumbo toilet paper rolls with 2,000 sheets which are generally used in public restrooms.[53]

"Y2K and The Great Hawaiian Toilet Paper Panic" During the oil embargo situation of the mid-1970's, Hawaii went into widespread pandemonium. Since all of Hawaii's sources are being shipped from 6,000 miles away to the state, the shipping "interruption" caused a huge disturbance to Hawaii's people. The store shelves were lacking in many areas, but the paper product department was getting the worst end of the deal. The toilet paper had to be rationed out once a new shipment came in, one roll per person only.[69] Just like this year (2020]

Toilet Paper Q&A

How much time does a person spend on the toilet over a lifetime? According to various studies, the average person spends 3 years on the toilet over the course of a lifetime![231] I probably spent this much time on the toilet just as a child.

How often do people urinate and defecate? People typically have a bowel movement at least once every 24 hours. People urinate on average 6 times a day.[87] Using my bidet I defecate 2-3 times most every day, sometimes more.

How many days does the standard roll of toilet paper last in a household bathroom? According to Charmin customers, the number of days a standard roll of bath tissue usually lasts in the most-used bathrooms in the house is five.[69]

What is the average number of toilet tissue sheets a person uses in one day? On average, consumers use 8.6 sheets per trip – a total of 57 sheets per day. That's an annual total of 20,805 sheets![69]

How did late-nighter Johnny Carson create to the Great Toilet Paper Shortage of 1973? It all actually started as a joke. Johnny Carson's quote: "You know what's disappearing from the supermarket shelves? Toilet paper. There's an acute shortage of toilet paper in the United States." The next morning, many of the 20 million television viewers ran to the supermarket and bought all of the toilet paper they could find. By noon, most of the stores were out of stock! Carson later apologized for scaring the public, and retracted his quote.[69,120]

"What is your toilet paper preference? Mine is the one that is most comfortable." "It's like fine wine, there are many selections and many are excellent." – Kenn Fischburg, author of Toilet Paper Encyclopedia.[119]

What FACTORS of TP are important in public restrooms?
• Tissue texture – 75%
• Softer paper – 36%
• Not running out of paper – 31%

• Toilet paper with moisturizer – 13% [69]

How much tissue/tissue products are produced each year? According to the American Forest & Paper Association, approximately 5.8 million tons of tissue grades, consisting of toilet and facial tissue, paper napkins, towels, diapers, and various other sanitary products are produced in the U.S. annually. In 1992, approximately 3.5 million tons of scrap paper was used to manufacture these products.[53]

How is toilet paper ranked in popularity among mass merchandisers? Across the food, drug and mass merchandiser outlets, bathroom tissue is ranked third among all non-food product categories.[53]

What is wet-strength? Normally, paper loses most of its strength when saturated with water. A toilet tissue that retains more than 15% of its dry-strength when completely saturated with water may be correctly referred to as "wet-strength paper".[53]

What makes toilet paper soft? During the drying process, the toilet paper sheet is adhered to one large steel cylinder to dry and is then scraped (or "creped" off) by a metal blade. "Creping" imparts flexibility and stretch into the sheet, while lowering the strength and density, resulting in soft tissue products.[53]

What is Toilet Paper (TP)?

Tissue is a general term indicating a class of papers of characteristic gauzy texture, and in some cases, fairly transparent. Tissue papers are made on any type of paper machine, from any type of pulp, including reclaimed paper stock. They may be glazed, unglazed, or creped, and are used for a variety of purposes. Examples are primarily sanitary grades such as toilet, facial, napkin, toweling, wipes, and special sanitary papers. Desirable characteristics are softness, strength, and freedom from lint.[53]

Over the ages human beings have employed various methods of personal cleansing following urination and defecation, including leaves, rags, seaweed, straw, grass, snow, sand, corncobs, coconut shells, newspapers, and in particular catalog pages. Those with means enjoyed relative comfort and luxury: French royalty used lace, while hemp served upper class needs in many cultures and rosewater-infused wool was prized in ancient Rome. Defecating in running bodies of water was considered an efficient method of washing, and disposing of waste and still is in some developing areas. Increasingly the method of choice for many individuals worldwide is toilet paper. There is virtually nowhere on the planet where toilet paper is not used, at least occasionally.[48]

Kenaf yields (for paper) are 7-15 times greater than wood obtained from managed natural northern forests (whenharvested on a 50-year cycle). Recorded yields for annually harvested kenaf, for instance, are about 2.4 times those of plantation-grown southern yellow pine harvested on a faster 20-year cycle.[293]

Toilet paper, sometimes called toilet tissue in Britain, is a tissue paper product primarily used to clean the anus and surrounding area of fecal material after defecation and to clean the perineal area of urine after urination or other bodily fluid releases. It also acts as a layer of protection for the hands during these processes. It is usually supplied as a long strip of perforated paper wrapped around a paperboard core for storage in a dispenser near a toilet.[2]

Procter & Gamble enjoyed success marketing Wet Wipes as a replacement or follow-up for toilet paper. Today, these damp cloth wipes have grown into a $2.2 billion industry. The market is so massive that it has inspired three male-targeted wipes, Bro Wipes, Dude Wipes, and One Wipe Charlies, which position themselves as testosterone-fueled counterparts to feminized bidets and hygiene products. They have even popped up in music, including a rap song by Cam'ron in which the chorus—"Go get ya wet wipes"—is a prompt for freshening up before sex.[68]

There is a growing number of families who use a toilet cloth (commonly called "family cloth") instead of tissue, sometimes using a portable spray bottle for their primary wash. I do not see much difference between this and using a bidet.

Once reserved for Europeans, bidets are now popular all over the world—except in North America. Thomas reports that 60 percent of Japanese households today have high-tech bidets made by Toto called Washlets.[20]

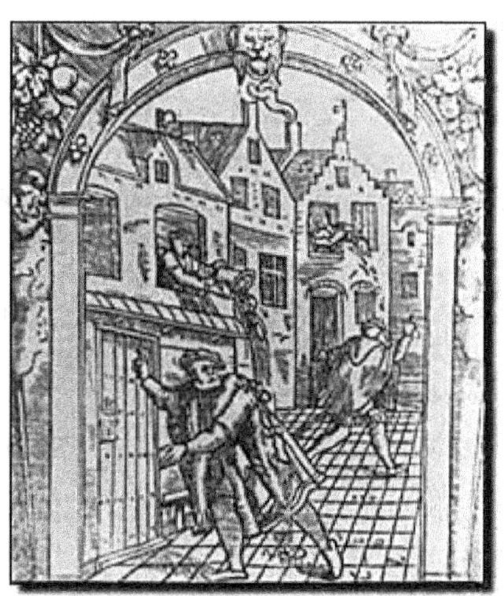

TP Economics

What's your impression of the tissue category [asking a Major buyer, 2019]?" "We follow pulp prices very closely, since it has such a high influence on our costs. And it's been flying high recently, rising from about $900 to over $1200 for NBSK (the benchmark grade, northern bleached softwood kraft)".[250]

Basically, the huge industry of producing toilet paper could be eliminated through the use of bidets.[20]

Economics comes from two Latin words basically meaning "home management". How are we managing our Earth home? There is no doubt that our paper industry is a major employer, makes a lot of money, and is one of our best export markets. The profits made and the wages earned do not offset huge environmental costs that are spiraling out of control. We may never be able to offset these costs. Paper production, especially tissue, has continued to grow unabated since the first edition of this book. What was then alarming, is now terrifying. The number of trees being cut down in the world for paper is not sustainable, and is actually endangering our continued existence on this earth. Nor do we have enough water to make enough TP for even most of the world, nor enough water for everyone to flush their waste.

Gene quotes **The Humanure Handbook**, "It takes between 1000 and 2000 tons of water at various stages in the process to flush one ton of humanure. In a world of just six billion people producing a conservative estimate of 1.2 metric tons of human excrement daily, the amount of water required to flush it all would not be obtainable".[270]

Economic Costs of TP Production
System Costs

Finding any data on the economic costs of producing TP was incredibly difficult, and even worse much data has disappeared since the first edition. The figures can vary greatly from one source to another, so I have tried to show the general range. Establishing consistent dates for this data was virtually impossible to obtain.

World TP production: 83-100 million rolls a day.[6,231]

US Tot use of TP (annually): near 12 billion rolls.[231]

$TP US purchases (2005): $5.7 billion a year.[239]

$TP US purchases (2018): $10.9 billion a year.[232]

$TP US tissue sales: $31 billion a year.[225]

$Gr Sales all paper: $200 billion annually.[53]

Water to mfg US TP: 473,587,500,000 gallons a year.[87,187]

US chlorine used (annually): 253,000 tons a year.[20]

US electricity used: 17,300,000,000 KW hours a year.[20]

Water used per roll TP: between 12-37 gallons.[20,87]

Electricity used per roll TP: 1.3 Kilowatt hours.[20]

(enough to power our house for a day)

Avg. US flush: 4 gallons per flush.[20]

Avg. US bidet flush: .125 gallons per flush.[20]

US ton recycled TP benefits: saves 24,000 gallons water.[48]

US ton recycled TP benefits: 3,000 - 4,000 kWh electricity saved.[55]

US ton recycled TP benefits: 74% less air pollution.[48]

US ton recycled TP benefits: saves 17 trees.[48]

US ton recycled TP benefits: creates 5+ more jobs.[48]

Paper can be recycled: 6 times (each time the fibers get shorter).[55]

US Virgin fiber used (2005): 3,113,000 metric tons a year.[58]

US Boreal virgin fiber use (K-C): 435,820 metric tons.[58]

Canada Boreal loss 1996-2015: >28 million acres.[225] (size of Ohio)

TP lifetime use one individual: 384 trees.[231,242]

US paper cups consumed (2006) annually: 16 billion cups annual.[271]

US paper cups consumed (2006) annually: 4 billion gal. of water.[271]

US paper cups consumed (2006) annually: 253 million pounds of waste.[271]

US paper cups consumed (2006) annually: 6.5 million trees/year.[271]

US paper cups consumed (2006) annually: 4 billion gallons.[271]

US paper cups consumed (2006) annually: 253 million pounds of waste.[271]

Municipal Sewage Systems

Plumbing infiltration has improved dramatically from just 60 years ago; back in 1950 one fourth of the country and over 50% of rural residents lacked complete plumbing facilities.[122]

[France 1700s?] A number of enactments, however, could not prevent people to defecate in the open. A delegation led by master weaver protested in front of the French Municipal Building and said, "Our fathers have defecated at the place where you prevent us to do. We have defecated here and now our children will defecate there"... At the same time, there was no hesitation in letting loose pigs to eat human excreta.[7]

Besides flush-toilets relatively unquestioned social integration, it is their complexity as an infrasystem that is comprised of a series of social and physical components that are regulated by public, private, and possibly informal institutions as a means to create, maintain, and improve a sanitation infrastructural service. Flush-toilets are one component or interface within a sanitation system necessitating to some degree a series of sewer mains, feeder pipes, pumps, different pressure systems, and drainage along with a series of different water and waste treatment systems.[234]

Flush-toilets, despite their benefits, have serious drawbacks in terms of health, environmental sustainability, and operation. Despite the undeniable benefits of flush-toilets, there is also a surreptitious aspect constructed into

104

these instillations and piping infrastructures. This paper argues, despite the real material benefits administered by flush-toilets, that it nevertheless contributes to infrastructural and structural violence through the industrialized degradation of the natural environment, while maintaining and accelerating the existing relationship of the industrial economy along with the establishment of human dependency and bodily atrophy. These negative outcomes associated with flush-toilets stem principally from their function and composition within the globalized industrial economy.[234]

I could not find any costs for building a modern municipal sewage system, but the costs of fixing New Jersey's system alone will cost billions of dollars.[260] The costs of a household septic system are currently estimated at between $3,072 and $9,087.[261] One estimate to develop an industrial sewage facility (that then connects with a municipal sewage system) appears to be $460,000 each.[262] There are additional costs for feeder lines, reservoirs, leach fields, etc. One county had to scrap its plan to simply extend it's sewer system because it would cost at least $35 milion.[264]

The oldest archeological discovery of working toilets dates back to 3000 BC Scotland. In their Neolithic settlement Skara Brae scientists found remnants of the stone huts, fully equipped with drains that extended from the recesses in the walls. This extremely early and very sophisticated example of toilet technology was not seen in other more advanced cultures for thousands of years, managing even to remain superior to any design in entire world.[53]

The vast majority of the 80 percent of Americans who don't use septic tanks are served by municipal water-treatment plants. Waste from their homes is whisked immediately off the premises, never to be seen, smelled, or considered again. Pipes carry waste from these homes to wastewater-treatment plants that, in some ways, work like a septic tank on a very large scale.[259]

New Jersey's cities face a multi-billion-dollar price tag to fix combined sewer systems that dump more then 23 billion gallons of raw sewage into our waterways every year. The cost of not fixing them will be even higher. In a combined sewer system, when the combined volume of sewage and storm water is too great for the treatment plant to handle, the system is designed, quite deliberately, to discharge them directly into nearby water bodies without treatment. These combined sewer overflows (CSOs) pollute rivers and bays during rain events. CSOs additionally can cause sewer backups into basements and streets, threatening human health. They have a significant environmental impact, causing closure of beaches and shellfish beds and impairing fish and other aquatic life and their habitats.[260]

History of toilets spans our entire modern history, but widespread adoption of public and private bathrooms started to appear only in the last 500 years, powered by the rising tide of invention, technology and industry.[53]

Home Septic Systems

Septic tank owners (about 20 percent of Americans) are most likely to be able to give an accurate answer to the cost of ownership of a home septic system, because they're responsible for the maintenance of their own sewage-disposal systems. A flush from one of their toilets sends wastewater to a tank buried on their property, where the waste products separate into solid and liquid layers and partially decompose. The liquid layer flows out of the tank and into a drain field that disperses it into the soil, where naturally occurring microbes remove harmful bacteria, viruses, and nutrients. The solid layer stays behind in the form of sludge that must be pumped out periodically as part of routine maintenance. If the tank is properly designed and maintained, those bacteria, viruses, and nutrients stay out of groundwater and surface water that people may use for drinking water, and they never reach surface water bodies where people swim or boat.[259]   In addition, some brands of wipes contain alcohol, which can kill the bacteria and enzymes responsible for breaking down solid waste in septic tanks.[253]

There have been improvements to septic tank technology over the years, yet many tanks are like my own that is at least 50 years old! Our is doing quite well, but there's bound to me many septic system that are nothing more than cesspools oozing sewage into streams or into the yard grass or the nearby road ditch. Gene once asked a health inspector once how many such cesspool septic tanks were still operating and he said, "You don't want to go there." Neither do many of the owners of those leaking cesspools; there is no incentive to identify, or money to fix them in poor rural counties.[270]

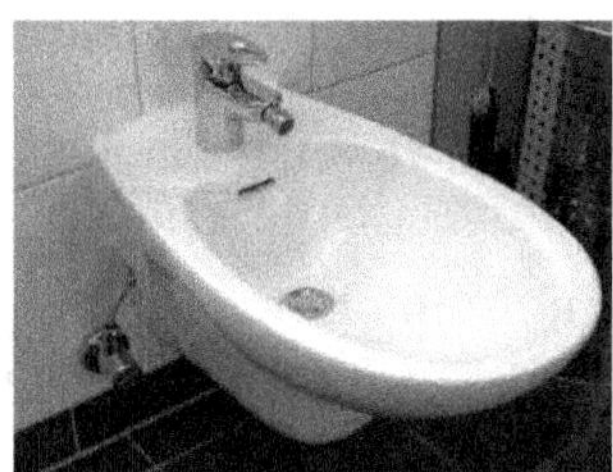

Clogged Plumbing

What are the costs of flushing toilet paper, aside from major environmental costs? Clogged drains, both in your own home and in your city. Bidets greatly reduce the level of waste material in the city sewage systems and treatment plants and can also minimize the chance of clogs in your own home plumbing system - which are frequently caused by toilet paper blockages (or worse, wet wipes). If you have a septic system as we do, there is the added expense of having someone periodically empty your storage tank largely because of the accumulated paper. To be fair, we personally have had to empty our septic system only once in 45 years, and much of the residue was from the former owners.[28,270]

In medieval Europe lavatories took several forms, but they were very rare. Mostly they were created over castle or village motes, suspended in air with simple wooden buildings or in castle galleries. Waste that fell in those motes served as excellent repellant to enemy forces who wanted to enter into the city by force, but sadly such waste attracted many diseases.[53]

Many people buy wipes for their convenience. Wet Wipes are relatively cheap to buy, but their disposal costs are immense and increasing daily. Wet Wipes have clogged innumerable home septic systems, often necessitating the expense of plumbers to clean up the mess. They've created major damage to sewer systems from Los Angeles to London. Once flushed, the wipes can glom together with any fat from food waste and can form what are called "fatbergs"—iceberg-style blockages that can totally "stop up" a city's sewer system. To extract a fatberg and make the needed repairs can be incredibly pricey; in London back in 2015, one 10-ton fatberg cost the city $600,000. And last September, the city discovered another that's approximately 140 tons, which could very well cost 10 times as much to remove.[68,252-3]

Always ensure any wipes you use are indeed flushable. We get an awful lot of blocked toilet calls from people flushing wipes down the toilet - Ray Green.[69]

I work in the waste water industry. I can tell you firsthand that these wipes are a menace. They will clog up your home plumbing. When they do make it into the public sewer system they wreak havoc with the pumps at the pumping stations. I spend most of my day pulling flushable wipes out of pumps they have clogged. If not gotten to in time, clogged pumps at a pump station can cause an overflow which is a public health hazard. Flushable? Yes. Non-clogging? No. Biodegradable? Perhaps over time but not before they cause the aforementioned problems.[69]

Personal Economy

Finally, consider how much money we spend on medications for our sore or chafed anus and genital area, for constipation, for diarrhea, and so on, that would be ameliorated by the use of a bidet. We should also include a certain amount of what we spend on infections originating in this area as well. Plus time lost from work; I have no figures on this but it should be a significant sum. On top of that is significant personal inconvenience (at least). If using a bidet eliminates even a good percentage of these expenses, we will have some real personal economy and better national health.

Americans have a new favorite way to flush money down the drain: luxury toilet paper. Sales in the United States of what the industry calls "luxury" rolls — anything quilted, lotioned, perfumed or ultra-soft, from two- to four-ply — climbed to $1.4 billion last year, outpacing all other kinds of toilet paper for the first time in nearly a decade.[249]

The New York Times reported a 40% increase in sales of luxury brands of toilet paper in 2008. Paper companies are anxious to keep those percentages up, even as the recession bites. And Reuters reported that Kimberly-Clark spent $25m in its third quarter on advertising to persuade Americans against trusting their bottoms to cheaper brands (2009).[56,266]

The struggle for toilet paper chains is convincing shoppers that pricier luxury papers aren't just flushing cash down the toilet. Even during a recession, analysts said, they saw shoppers who were more than willing to trade up for one of the few indulgences they could afford. "Even in a down market, people want a little bit of luxury," Umphress said. "They may not be able to take a spa vacation. But they can make their home a little bit more spa-like".[249]

• 84% of households buy Premium and Super Premium brand toilet paper
• 64% of households buy Regular and Economy brand toilet paper
• 48% of households buy all four categories! [119]

Industry Profit

As often happens with the introduction of a new innovation, the harmful environmental consequences of the use of toilet paper were not taken into consideration when this method of cleansing was adopted. Given the ongoing wide scale consumption of this product, one might suggest this is still the case. Toilet paper is a product with a very short one-time-use lifespan and every day an equivalent of 27,000 trees is flushed down the toilet worldwide. Harmful chemicals like dioxin or phosphorus are some of the by-products from the production process... Over the last years, the consumption of toilet paper is growing on a global scale. [66]

I am not a fan of our corporate system that values profit over everything else. This is exemplified by the very profitable paper industry. They have the resources and money to make TP a truly sustainable product, but haven't, yet.

Between 1980 and 2004 annual market consumption grew from 1 billion rolls to 2.7 billion rolls. the increase fuelled primarily by a combination of population growth and increased per capita consumption. [244]

Procter & Gamble enjoyed success marketing (wipes) as a replacement or follow-up for toilet paper. Today, these damp cloth wipes have grown into a $2.2 billion industry. [68]

The U.S. tissue market generates $31 billion in revenue every year, second only to China. [225] Americans who make up just over 4 percent of the world's population, are still the big spenders. We account for about 20 percent of global tissue consumption. [225] US consumers spent $5.7 billion on TP back in 2005. [239]

Pulp Mill Watch, a website sponsored by the German nonprofit Urgewald, projected that by 2012 the pulp industry would expand production by over 25 million tons, fed by monoculture plantations established in Australia, Brazil, China, Indonesia, Russia, South Africa, Thailand, and Uruguay, primarily to feed the market demand for virgin toilet paper in North America and Europe. [48]

Globally, tissue is the fastest-growing sector in the paper industry and is expected to grow almost 6 percent annually from 2018 to 2022. Americans remain among their most voracious consumers. [225]

But it is the international industry giant driving the market-a global market it claims is clamoring for the softest, most absorbent, thickest toilet paper, which can only be manufactured from virgin fiber. And while it is true that the source of fiber for many tissue products is wood waste created in other segments of the wood industry, the fact remains that there is no strong movement among many toilet tissue companies to shift consumer preferences to more environmentally friendly products-although, it is interesting to note, these same consumers regularly use recycled-content toilet paper on the road, at sporting events, and at work. [48]

How important is tissue for Kroger? For us, it's huge, because it's a very essential item that has super-high household penetration rates. It drives customers to our stores and that's very important. And as far as our own spending to buy the products we sell, tissue is certainly one of the bigger spends that we have, so there is more focus on that category.[251]

"What's your impression of the tissue category?" "Tissue is a very exciting business. Every day you're hearing about new developments, so it's a very dynamic category. Of course, if you are standing outside the tissue category, you would think that paper is just paper, and it's very simple. But it certainly isn't. Once you get into the details you realize it's very complicated. There are many important variables such as sheet counts, plies, basis weight, softness, strength, pulp qualities, and all the different technologies that can be used to give these products the properties we are searching for. Those complexities were attractive to me, because I like something that's challenging and makes me hungry to know more".[251]

Paper manufacturers such as Kimberly-Clark have identified luxury brands such as three-ply tissues or tissues infused with hand lotion as the fastest-growing market share in a highly competitive industry. Its latest television advertisements show a woman caressing tissue infused with hand lotion. Dave Dixon, a company spokesman, said toilet paper and tissue from recycled fiber had been on the market for years. If Americans wanted to buy them, they could (though I certainly can't find them in Willits)... but "It's [not] the quality and softness the consumers in America have come to expect."... Reuters reported that Kimberly-Clark spent $25m in its third quarter on advertising to persuade Americans against trusting their bottoms to cheaper brands.[266]

The New York Times reported a 40% increase in sales of luxury brands of toilet paper in 2008. Paper companies are anxious to keep those percentages up, even as the recession bites. And Reuters reported that Kimberly-Clark spent $25m in its third quarter on advertising to persuade Americans against trusting their bottoms to cheaper brands (2009).[56,266]

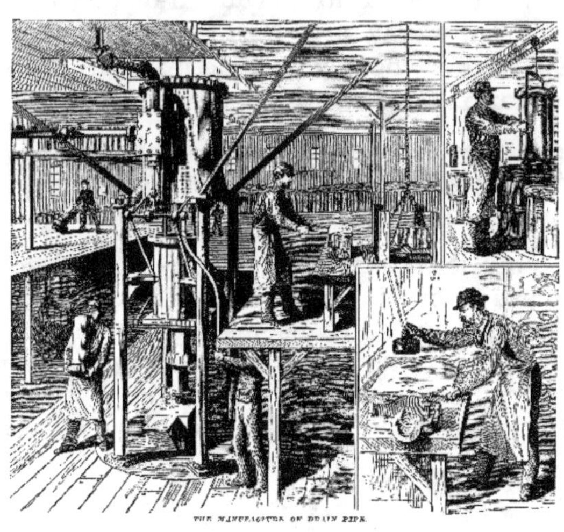

Social Economic Costs

For the last 40 centuries, toilets and sanitation systems utilized feces as a useable resource; a concept now lost with the hygiene and flush-toilet infrasystems in use today. Common in China, Korea, and Japan were aquaculture toilets that placed latrines over fishponds in order to farm fresh water fish (tilapia) and plants (macrophyls) such as water spinach and mimosa as they thrived in feces-contaminated waters. The pot-toilet was an outhouse that collected stools in a pot which would later be composted for agricultural fertilizer... public toilets were constructed and supported by farmers as they were a means to harvest human excrement for agricultural purposes. These systems are notable for their ability to turn what was later considered a waste into a resource—appreciating, utilizing, and interacting (in a responsible manner) with what would later become a taboo and morally condemned feature of the body with the rise of industrial capitalism, cities, and hygiene.[234]

Costs to Our Agriculture

Sim Van der Ryn, author of **The Toilet Papers**, references a 1974 report pointing out that Los Angeles at that time was dumping about 235 million gallons of primary treated effluent and 100 million gallons of secondary effluent into the ocean every day. "It got me to thinking, " Sim writes, "the nutrients in all that effluent, much of it from flush toilets, if converted to fertilizer, would be the equivalent of 200 tons of 7-14-12 fertilizer... Each ton when applied to soil would provide the nutrients to grow 25 tons of vegetables. Sim figures each day, L.A.'s waste provides the nutrients to grow 5000 tons of vegetables, enough to provide everyone in Los Angeles with a pound or two of fresh produce daily.[270]

Strikingly in the 1860s, Professor Justus von Liebig warned that "the introduction of water flush closets into most parts of England results in the annual loss of the materials capable of producing food for three and a half million people," suggesting sewage should not be discharged into rivers, but integrated into an agricultural systems on the outskirts of cities.[234]

The boy asks him what he's going to do with all that cow poop. The man says, "I'm taking it home to put on my strawberries." The little boy looks up at the man and says, "I don't know where you come from sir, but where I come from we put cream and sugar on our strawberries".[298]

I am indebted to Gene Logsdon and his book, **Holy Shit, Managing Manure to Save Mankind**, for some of the information in this section. I strongly recommend that you read this book. It is hilarious, sobering, and educational.

Over the last two centuries, cheap manufactured fertilizers and a seemingly unlimited acreage have allowed the United States to become the champion wastrel of the world. One can only imagine the famine and chaos that would result if we tried to continue that kind of extravagance for forty centuries. As sources of chemical fertilizers decline, either manure will once more become the pot of gold at the end of the rainbow or population level will dramatically decline.[270]

As part of Ecology Action over the past thirty years we were acutely aware that our doom from "peak oil" was nothing compared to "peak water" and "peak potash". This is not on the radar of our highly urbanized society which sees agriculture as dirty business best ignored. We got tired of crying wolf but the wolf is truly at our door. We have good reason to believe that the era of reliance on manufactured and mined fertilizer is passing. Modern industrialized agriculture is completely dependent on cheap chemical fertilizers and has largely forgotten any other way.

By making full use of animal wastes Asian farmers have been one of the few agricultural systems to remain productive and fertile for hundreds of years. Logsdon mentions that in 1907 Asian farmers were sustainably harvesting five times what American farmers were producing. Even today only intensive gardening methods like biointensive gardening can approach these yields sustainably. Back then if they didn't keep production up people starved. Will we be faced with starvation if we do not start getting our shit together?[270]

What happens when we do run out of cheap fertilizers? Such as the world supply of agricultural phosphorus is running dangerously low. So much so that phosphorus has been listed among the "endangered elements" where there is a risk to future supply. Scientists predict a world shortage within about 30 to 40 years. Hennig Brand found phosphorus in buckets of urine 350 years ago; how interesting that this is still the best place to find it today.[310]

This points to the need to develop phosphorus recycling, ideally at the point before it becomes highly diluted in our water streams. So how could this be done? Humans consume 3m tons more phosphorus than they need each year, which is eventually excreted as urine and faeces. Recycling phosphorus from human waste might not sound a very uplifting endeavour, but it will be a golden egg for whoever finds a way to do it.[310]

Getting all the manure and other organic wastes needed to maintain yields high enough to support rising populations without a full complement of commercial fertilizers would be an enormous challenge requiring new agriculture and cultural attitudes.... The idea that all of agriculture might have to rely on animal (and human) waste to maintain the necessary soil fertility to keep the world from starving is not at all new to civilization. Only in the last hundred years or so has it been possible to lard enough anhydrous ammonia, superphosphate, and muriate of potash on crops to attain record-breaking yields (while burning and beating organic matter out of the soil). Before this "progress," human society has no other choice but to consider manure – animal and human – to be more precious than gold. At least humans did so in countries that sustained an ample food supply for long periods of time, as China and Japan did. We all need to read again Farmers of Forty Centuries by E. H. King, published in 1901, about Asian agriculture at that time. In Japan, Korea, and China, manure was treated like a precious gem because it was a precious gem. Every scrap of animal waste, human waste, and plant residue was scrupulously collected and reapplied to the land. So precious was manure that Chinese farmers stored it in burglar-proof containers. The polite thing to do after enjoying a meal at a friend's house was to go to the bathroom before you departed. I am not making that up.[270]

As I plow through the acres of figures pertaining to the amount of human excrement produced per year, and the costs involved in managing it, the most significant statistic to me is that humans discharge from their bodies something approaching 50 million tons of recoverable nitrogen, phosphorous, and potassium per year. That's not an easy figure to translate into monetary value, but let's just say that commercial fertilizer costs 50 cents a pound on average (a year or so ago it was higher, now it is lower, but all indications are that it is edging up again). We're talking $50 billion a year in biosolid fertilizer that we are mostly throwing away, after spending incalculable amounts of money to do the throwing. That is a lot of cash, even for these speculative times. Surely that's enough incentive to attract researchers, entrepreneurs, and innovative companies into developing a way to keep human sludge separated from the industrial and household contaminants that go down the sewer drains with it.[270]

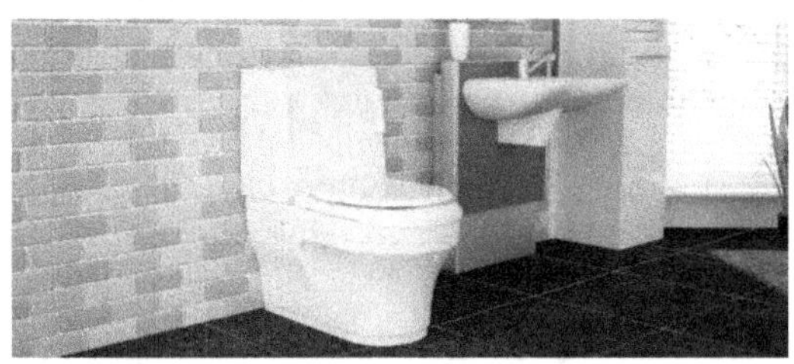

Costs To Our Forests

Deforestation is one of the major contributing factors to global climate change. NRDC says that while toilet tissue accounts for only 15 percent of deforestation, any industry focused on virgin wood products - whether from boreal forests or plantations - is culpable. "Virgin fiber is not the optimal fiber source for disposable tissue products," says Allen Hershkowitz of NRDC. "Instead, disposable tissue products should be made from recycled fibers, which avoids forestry impacts entirely".[48]

When future historians cast around for symbols of our current age of consumerism, I reckon they'll be hard pressed to go past toilet paper. "For centuries, billions of humans cleansed themselves after defecation using a soft, paper product made from trees," could well be the introduction to the year 2497 (digital) bestseller "What Went Wrong?" Kiddo, we used to have these things called trees.[230]

One of the earliest surviving works of literature, the 4000-year-old Sumerian Epic of Gilgamesh tells the story of a powerful Mesopotamian king who sets out on an adventure to find not treasure but trees because his city has so little wood with which to build.[230]

For example, of Australia's forests standing at the time of European settlement in 1788, 40 per cent have already been cleared, 35 per cent have been partly logged, and only 25 per cent remain intact, with logging continuing in old growth forests.[230]

In 2005 the Food and Agriculture Organization (FAO) of the United Nations, which monitors the state of the world's forests every few years, reported that 13 million hectares of global forests are lost annually, including 6 million hectares of what are described as primary forests-some of the most biologically diverse ecological systems in the world. And although ongoing depletion of forests in the Amazon is a focus of environmental alarm, a 2009 report published in Trends in Ecology and Evolution detailed the escalating threat to boreal forests in Russia, Alaska, Canada, and Scandinavia. According to the online magazine World Science, "the boreal, or northern forest, comprises about one-third of the world's forested area and one-third of the world's stored carbon." Canada's old growth and intact forests are logged at a rate of five acres a minute, 24 hours a day.[48]

Worldwide consumption of paper has risen by 400% in the past 40 years, with 35% of harvested trees being used for paper manufacture. Plantation forests, from where the majority of wood for pulping is obtained, is generally a monoculture and this raises concerns over the ecological effects of the practices.... Cutting down trees to make forest products such as pulp and paper creates temporary or long-term environmental disturbances in forest habitats depending on how carefully the harvest is carried out. There might be impacts on plant and animal biodiversity, soil fertility and water quality.[271]

Much of the tissue pulp in the United States comes from the boreal forest of Canada. This vast landscape of coniferous, birch, and aspen trees contains some of the last of the world's remaining intact forests, and is home to over 600 Indigenous communities, as well as boreal caribou, pine marten, and billions of songbirds. Yet, industrial logging claims more than a million acres of boreal forest every year. Many of the leading tissue companies in the United States stubbornly continue to rely on virgin fiber pulp in their flagship at - home tissue products rather than investing in existing alternatives.[225]

The global boreal is especially vital to worldwide efforts to fight climate change since it stores more carbon per hectare than any other forest biome on earth and holds more carbon than all the currently accessible oil, gas, and coal reserves combined. The Canadian boreal contains at least 12 percent of the world's carbon stores in its plants and soils. Every year, the Canadian boreal region, including peat lands, removes carbon dioxide equivalent to the annual emissions of 24 million passenger vehicles... Between 1996 and 2015, more than 28 million acres of boreal forest were logged, an area roughly the size of Ohio.[225] [Natural Defenses Defense Council, "The Issue With Tissue - How Americans are flushing forest down the toilet" (2019)]

Think about it. You and I can live up to two months without food, perhaps three days without water but only roughly five minutes with no oxygen. Despite this, the dominant global culture of the west insists we cut down one of our major sources of oxygen - trees - at a rate of 27,000 a day so even our most humble citizen may wipe their bottom. It's a rather perverse "f-you" to Mother Nature yet hardly the sole example of humanity's belligerent and systemic disdain for its well-being, nor of our cavalier attitude to trees.[230]

Basically, the huge industry of producing toilet paper could be eliminated through the use of bidets.20

Over 6.5 million trees were cut down to make 16 billion paper cups used by US consumers solely in 2006, using 4 billion US gallons (15,000,000 m3) of water and resulting in 253 million pounds of waste. Overall, North Americans use 58% of all paper cups, amounting to 130 billion cups.[271]

The worldwide adaptation of flush-toilets as a replacement for squatting toilets is driving the demand for toilet paper and even in countries that prefer wet sanitation (i.e. cleaning with water) over dry sanitation (i.e. cleaning with paper) like Indonesia and India. The exposure to AFH (i.e. away from home) flush-toilets and toilet paper has led to an increased popularity of toilet paper.[66]

It appears that the consumption of toilet paper will be a continuing global need as population growth adds to the over 2 billion people currently estimated to be lacking access to sanitation.[48]   About four billion people don't use toilet paper. About 70%-75 % of the world's population does not use toilet paper.[53]

Toilet and tissue paper, now increasingly used by Indians even though they are both disgustingly unhealthy, account for 1 per cent of the total paper consumption. Between 1978 and 1987 paper production in India went up by 91 per cent, while in the rest of the world it went up by 39 per cent. Between 1987 up to now, we have gone up by another 100 per cent while world averages have gone even lower than 30 per cent... Use less paper. Otherwise, forget forests and animals, your life and mine. You will have exchanged your life for toilet paper. Maneka Gandhi.[227]

Sarah Bell, a water systems lecturer at University College London, pointed out in an email, "In India, more people have access to mobile phones than toilets. In some parts of the world it is easier to share cat videos on Facebook than it is to find a safe place to do a poo. That's completely nuts".[27]

What Kimberly-Clark Should Do: Maximize post-consumer recycled and agricultural residue fiber content: Stop producing tissue products that are manufactured solely out of virgin wood fibers. Maximize post-consumer recycled content and/or fiber from agricultural residues in all tissue products. Minimize fiber requirements by redesigning products and increasing production efficiency. Stay out of endangered forests: Stop using wood fiber from the Canadian boreal and other endangered forests. Stop buying pulp or wood fiber from operations that use environmentally unsustainable forestry practices, such as converting natural forests to plantations or clear cutting. Ensure that any virgin wood fiber it uses comes from sustainable logging operations that are certified to Forest Stewardship Council standards. For more information on the Forest Stewardship Council please visit www.fsc.org.[212]

China has set its sights on the global toilet paper market, aiming to become both the biggest consumer and producer of fine toilet tissue within the next decade.[117] China also correlates increased use of toilet paper with advancements in sanitation and improved health outcomes.[48]

As conceived in the West, the toilet is the first place outside of bed where one begins one's day and the last place before bed when ending the evening.[8] (not quote, reported in [204])

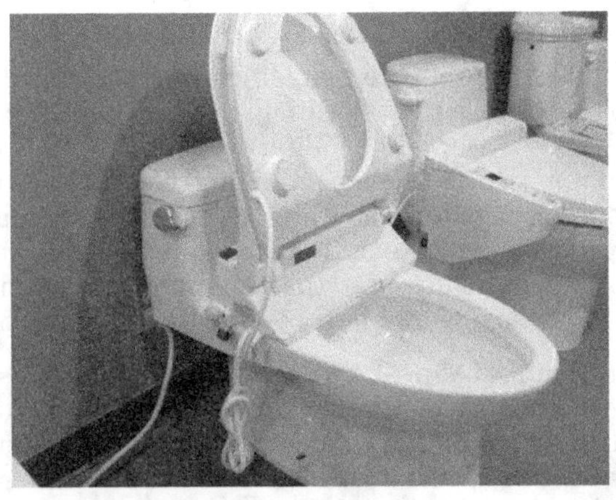

TP Environment

If you are reading this book, you most likely were raised on flush toilets and a municipal sewage system. This is ubiquitous in our society, we assume its constant presence where ever we are, and are upset if it isn't in place and working. We utterly depend on it, but it is all but unconscious.

As Pogo would say, "We have found the enemy, and it is us!" The United States is by far the biggest user (and producer, and waste-r) of tissue paper, and the damage we do to the world environment wiping our butts is pretty mind-boggling. Read on for the facts!

First of all, getting the facts on environmental damage caused by TP was very difficult. The data that two bidet websites offered in my first edition has disappeared in the ensuing 15 years. One would think that the ecological aspects of commercial paper making would be public knowledge, but in reality it is a closely guarded secret (unless you are willing to pay thousands of dollars for industry information). I felt like I was assaulting the CIA for classified information; and the payoff was incredibly scary! The sheer size of these numbers boggles the mind!

Fifteen years ago my first edition pointed out the statistics in this chapter, pointed out the huge ecological benefits of using a bidet, both personally and as a nation, and as a result eliminating most of our need for toilet paper. These pages now reveal that the continued growth in the use of toilet paper (and other tissue products) is quickly and inevitably destroying our world ecology. Turning to the bidet is perhaps our last chance at salvation.

In 2001 Americans were producing up to 100,000,000 rolls of toilet paper a day.[6] This amounts to 36,000,000,000 rolls of toilet paper produced per year, just in the US. In the US we use between 3.2 million tons-9.2 million tons of TP every year.[48,225]   That is 15 million trees a year pulped into TP, and the number is growing.[20]

Justin Thomas, editor of the website metaefficient.com, considers bidets to be "a key green technology" because they eliminate the use of toilet paper. According to his analysis, Americans use 36.5 billion rolls of toilet paper every year, representing the pulping of some 15 million trees. Says Thomas: "This also involves 473,587,500,000 gallons of water to produce the paper and 253,000 tons of chlorine for bleaching." He adds that manufacturing requires about 17.3 terawatts of electricity annually and that significant amounts of energy and materials are used in packaging and in transportation to retail outlets.[20]

Worldwide, the equivalent of almost 270,000 trees is either flushed or dumped in landfills every day, according to Claude Martin of WWF (Worldwide Fund for Nature). Roughly 10 percent of that total is attributable to toilet paper. The result is that forests in both the global North and South are under assault by paper companies competing to fill what they insist is an inexhaustible consumer demand for, among other paper products, soft, fluffy toilet paper. The expanding global demand for toilet paper and the accompanying environmental effects of raw material sourcing and manufacturing are intensifying the focus on the source and production of tissue: virgin pulp or recycled?[48]

What other damage does wiping our derrieres do to our environment? We use 3.7 billion gallons of water every day just to make TP, which ends up contaminated in known and still unknown ways.[87]

The Kraft process is the most dominant chemical pulping process worldwide. The problem of kraft mill odor emitted from the sulphides in the white liquor in the initial pulping has long been an environmental and public relations issue for the pulp and paper industry. The kraft mill odor is caused predominantly by malodourous reduced sulphur compounds, or total reduced sulphur compounds namely, methyl mercaptan, dimethylsulphide, dimethyldisulphide and hydrogen sulphide.[269] I can no longer find any figures on the amount of sulfur used, but it is an essential part of the dominant Kraft process, which significantly pollutes both water and air.

Also 253,000 tons of chlorine was consumed.[20] Consider that chlorine, sulphur, and their chemical derivatives presumably end up somewhere in our environment.

At least 17,000,000,000 Kilowatt hours of electricity are consumed just to make TP. The EPA estimated this to be enough to power 1,579,045 homes for a year on average.[87,255]

Also refer to the statistics listed earlier at the beginning of Toilet Paper Economics.

Gene Logsdon is adamant that using a dry toilet can turn a family's human waste into pathogen-free fertilizer without composting. He claims if you could allow the feces to age in place two years, that would eliminate all potentially harmful pathogens (bacteria, viruses, and other organisms that can cause disease in humans) "and satisfy the demands of even the most paranoid among us".[270]

How much time does a person spend on the toilet over a lifetime? The average person spends 3 years on the toilet over the course of a lifetime! [69]

Threats To the Public

How can you resist big business? US Sales for all paper were $200 billion a year,[53] and $31 billion just for US TP sales.[225] Worldwide consumption of paper has risen by 400% in the past 40 years.[271] TP is a big industry in the U.S., Canada, and the world. We export a lot of TP. What can we do against such a profitable soft and fluffy danger?

The National Resources Defense Council reports: "The pulp and paper industry may contribute to more global and local environmental problems than any other industry in the world. Paper manufacturers reach deep into species-rich forests for virgin timber, razing trees, polluting waterways and destroying precious wildlife habitat. Pulp and paper mills that use virgin timber are major generators of hazardous air pollutants, including dioxins and other cancer-causing chemicals. And the industry is the third largest industrial emitter of global warming pollution".[217]

The pulp and paper industry is among the world's largest generators of toxic air and water pollutants and waste products. It is the third largest generator of global warming pollution, and those emissions are projected to increase 100 percent by 2020 (!). This industry is the world's largest user of fresh water and among the largest users of energy. And it destroys natural forests that are essential for clean air and water, the atmosphere's chemistry, wildlife habitat, indigenous cultures, spiritual inspiration and recreation. In North America the manufacture of tissue products has particularly dire environmental and social consequences.[71]

Toilet paper use has negative environmental implications for soil depletion, water contamination and human health. The negative environmental impacts associated with toilet paper seem to be increasing as a growing number of people are starting to use toilet paper instead of cleansing methods based on water.[66]

The paper industry is responsible for the release of persistent toxic pollutants like chlorine, mercury, lead and phosphorus into the environment, resulting in a legacy of health problems including cancers, nerve disorders and fertility problems. Chlorine bleaching has been particularly widespread and although there has been some progress in shifting away from the use of elemental chlorine for bleaching, the use of any chlorine-based chemicals at all can still result in dangerous pollution, because they are the building blocks of organochlorines, which include some of the most toxic compounds on earth, such as dioxins and furans.[60]

The remaining sludge will be filtered out and is usually sent to a landfill or recycled. Part of the chemicals that were in the toilet paper will remain in the sludge and contaminate the soil if stored/buried in a landfill. Also, more methane, a greenhouse gas with 23 times the heat trapping capacity of carbon dioxide, will be released during the breakdown of toilet paper in the landfill. After the removal of the sludge, the wastewater undergoes more chemical treatment to remove dissolved metals and other built up toxins. POPs will remain in the water (WHO, 2016).[66]

According to the U.S. EPA's Toxics Release Inventory, pulp and paper ranks fourth among U.S. manufacturing industries in the release of dioxin and dioxin-like compounds to the air, and third in releases of these chemicals to water.[60]

Dioxin is a POP (persistent organic pollutant), which means it has a high chemical stability (a half life of 7-11 years once absorbed by fat tissue) and thus accumulates in the body or the environment (WHO, 2016). Production processes like pulping and strengthening the paper can involve environmental hazards as well. Wastewater of a pulp and paper mill discharges materials such as nitrogen and phosphorus, which can cause or exacerbate the depletion of oxygen in water bodies, also known as eutrophication (Canadian EPA, 1991). The pulp and paper industry is also associated with emissions of heavy metals. In Canada for example, this industry is the third source of lead emissions to water (Environment and Climate Change Canada, 2016).[66]

Threats To Humans in the Industry

A significantly increased mortality was seen for diabetes mellitus and for secondary tumors of the lung and liver among the pulp and paper mill workers. Indications of excess risks were also found for obstructive lung disorders, pulmonary emboli, accidents, and pneumonia, as well as for malignant lymphomas, leukemia's, and cancer of the pancreas and stomach.[294]

RESULTS: There were 1,340 malignant cases out of 5,898 deaths. Total cancer mortality was not increased in either sulfate or sulfite mill workers, or by gender. Lung cancer mortality was increased among female workers, especially in paper production, but not among male workers. Exposure to wood dust and sulfur dioxide frequently exceeded occupational exposure limits. CONCLUSIONS: Female paper production workers had an increased mortality from lung cancer.[11]

Threats Caused By Our Municipal Waste Systems

We documented earlier (System Costs: Municipal Sewage Systems) that when we have municipal sewage we all have to be part of it, we are part of a package deal; everyone processes their human waste through one system managed (and controlled) by professionals. If our municipal system fails, it fails for everyone.

Municipal sewage has been very reliable until the tissue industry sabotaged it with new, even more unsustainable products: wet wipes, super-saturated TP, and such. The growing story of "fatbergs" is an excellent example. We the public, of course, are culpable in our exuberant acceptance of such products. Our aggregate purchases are funding this insanity.

Fatbergs became a problem in the 2010s in England, because of ageing Victorian sewers and the rise in usage of disposable (so-called flushable) cloths. Comprised not only of wet wipes and fat, fatbergs may contain other items that do not break apart or dissolve when flushed down the toilet, such as sanitary napkins, cotton buds, needles, condoms and food waste washed down kitchen sinks. Additionally grease and fat blockages can cause sanitary sewer overflows, in which sewage is discharged into the environment without treatment. In the United States, almost half of all sewer blockages are caused by grease.[305]

90% of medications consumed are excreted as urinary waste. Today's sewer systems have a high concentration of pharmaceutical drugs.[122]

No please not wipes. What happens is if you sewage pipe is not completely smooth the wipes will/can snag. I have had loads of blocked pipes because of this. and trust me power jetting your pipe is not cheap. stick with the paper stuff. Plumber Solihull.[69]

Since the mid-2000s, wet wipes such as baby wipes have become more common for use as an alternative to toilet paper in affluent countries, including the United States and the United Kingdom. This usage has in been encouraged by manufacturers, who have labeled some wet wipe brands as "flushable". Wet wipes, even "flushable" ones, when flushed down the toilet, have been known to clog internal plumbing, septic systems, and public sewer systems. The tendency for fat and wet wipes to cling together encourages the growth of the problematic obstructions in sewers known as 'fatbergs'. In addition, some brands of wipes contain alcohol, which can kill the bacteria and enzymes responsible for breaking down solid waste in septic tanks.[253]

Some of the large animal slaughter yards now generate as much waste as all the human sewage from a large metropolitan area, but somehow are largely exempt from handling and treating their sewage the way municipalities do.[270]

.Combined Sewers

Our sewer systems are seriously outdated and overloaded. Many large city systems were built over a hundred years ago as combined sewers. The EPA has called overflows from combined sewer systems "the largest category of our Nation's wastewater infrastructure that still need to be addressed.[259]

Combined sewers collect human waste, industrial waste, and storm water runoff into a single pipe for treatment and disposal. Pipes carry waste from these homes to wastewater-treatment plants that, in some ways, work like a septic tank on a very large scale. Most combined systems are concentrated in the older cities of the Northeast and the Great Lakes region, but they also exist in other older cities as far-flung as Atlanta, Memphis, and San Francisco. In other words, the systems that pose risks today happen to be the ones—state-of-the-art when they were built, but not today—that are in some of the biggest cities in America, which have a combined population of approximately 40 million people. In Hoboken, for example, some sewer lines date back to the Civil War. Common sense says that pipes that have been buried for a century and a half tend to leak. Over time, they also get clogged with debris or even congealed cooking oil, resulting in narrowed pipes that overflow even more easily. Another drawback are harmful algal blooms like the one that cost Toledo, Ohio, its drinking water recently, or fish kills like the one recently reported off Long Island.[259]

The much-discussed dead zone in the Gulf of Mexico is fed by phosphorus, nitrogen, and other contaminants found in the untreated sewage that, according to EPA estimates, flows out of America's treatment plants during the 23,000 to 75,000 sanitary-sewer overflows that happen per year… the same pollutants can be washed into surface water from agricultural land, industrial sites, and fertilized lawns dotted with pet waste, **but the 3 to 10 billion gallons of untreated waste released from our sewage-treatment plants per year cannot help but have an impact.** Specifically, they affect the water you swim in and the water you drink.[259]

Our Part in This

You know what really worries me? In 2005 when I wrote the first edition of this book we spent $5,700,000,000 on TP,[239] but we have since surged (splurged) to spend $10,900,000,000 billion a year – just for TP![232] And we are not even the big spenders, the latest figures state that China spent $15,000,000,000 on TP![224] My friends, this is not sustainable. **Ten billion dollars in the US just for TP – imagine what social good we could do with an extra $10 billion, just by not smearing our butts with paper.**

Sales in the United States of what the industry calls "luxury" rolls - anything quilted, lotioned, perfumed or ultra-soft, from two- to four-ply - climbed to $1.4 billion in 2014, says the Euromonitor International show. This segment is the fastest growing segment of industry.[231]

The tenderness of the delicate American buttock is causing more environmental devastation than the country's love of gas-guzzling cars, fast food or McMansions, according to green campaigners. At fault, they say, is the US public's insistence on extra-soft, quilted and multi-ply products when they use the bathroom.[266] "This is a product that we use for less than three seconds and the ecological consequences of manufacturing it from trees is enormous," said Allen Hershkowitz, a senior scientist at the Natural Resources Defence Council... "Future generations are going to look at the way we make toilet paper as one of the greatest excesses of our age... Making toilet paper from virgin wood is a lot worse than driving Hummers in terms of global warming pollution.. People just don't understand that softness equals ecological destruction...More than 98% of the toilet rolls sold in America comes from virgin wood," said Hershkowitz, "In Europe and Latin America, up to 40% of toilet paper comes from recycled products".[56]

Only 2% of American households buy recycled-fiber toilet paper, compared to 20% in Europe.[66] If every US household replaced just one roll of virgin fiber toilet paper with one made from 100% recycled fibers, 423,900 trees would be saved.[46]

In the last five years, tissue demand has accelerated rapidly in China. Tissue consumption in China is 7.5 times higher than it was 20 years ago and annual volume growth has more than doubled to between 400,000-500,000 tons within less than 10 years. In fact, China is expected to account for close to 40% of global tissue growth in the coming years.[222]

As excessive as our consumption of TP is, the fact that China and other parts of the world are greatly expanding their consumption of TP is insanely scary. The world is adopting our flush system when the world ecology simply cannot support this system for everyone. There is not enough water or trees to fill everyone's need if the whole world is flushing TP down toilets. We have lost control over the spread of TP, and that is not good.

So how do we get to these inconceivable numbers? A few sheets of TP at a time. People typically have a bowel movement at least once every 24 hours. People urinate on average 6 times a day. It takes 5 gallons of water to flush the average American toilet. What happens when 7 billion people try to flush? (A bidet uses a pint of water on average).[87]

Bidets eliminate the need for toilet paper. Bidets pay for themselves very quickly over time; they also reduce a huge amount of pollution. Bidets result in using much less water, and we also have much less water badly polluted. If we all just use less toilet paper (better yet none at all!), our world and our environment will benefit greatly. If we don't, we will just go slowly into our collective demise.

And unlike most of his countrymen — or his wife, who balked at the price of the model the couple ended up buying for $1,248 — he was immediately smitten. Now, after 15 months of regular use, both Falsettis are ardent fans of the Washlet. "It sounds crazy," Mr. Falsetti said, "that you could like a toilet bowl seat so much".[38]

Toilet paper tends to break down in about eight seconds. In contrast, flushable wipes lasted well beyond 30 minutes and have been involved in numerous numerous cases of stopped-up sewer lines.[69] We have already read about some of the dangers of flushable wipes in **Toilet Paper Ecology**.

Flushable wipes have become very popular, but they might not be so popular in your septic system. These flushable wipes performed very poorly in their disintegration tests and may damage or back up your sewer or septic system.[69]

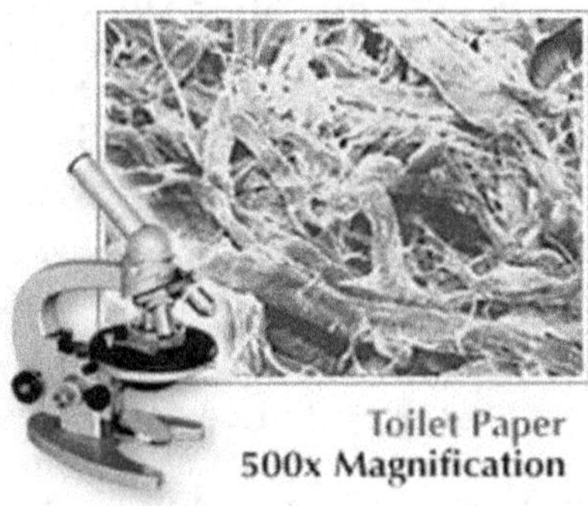

TP Un-Health

I have poked my fingers through TP into my defecation hundreds, maybe thousands of times (when I still used toilet paper). At times I thought there was no other way. I was often faced with the unpleasant option of wadding up an unconscionable amount of TP to get the job done, or almost certainly befouling my hand. I have always found TP in any form to be marginal for cleaning my derriere, even without soiling my fingers. TP is marginal for most any cleaning purpose in my experience. That, in essence, was the genesis of this book.

The industrial process of creating white TP involves the use of huge amounts of toxic chemicals, most of which end up in our environment (air, water or landfill). The two worst byproducts are dioxin (dioxine) and bisphenol A (BPA) which have their own sections below.

[This "post hygiene" wash liquid was allowed to fall into a sterilized basin and was subsequently transferred to a sterile Erlenmeyer flask, removed to a laboratory, and evaluated for the presence of micro-organisms. The number of bacteria in the post-hygiene TSB wash signifies the efficacy of the personal hygiene step; that is, the lower the bacteria numbers in the post-hygiene wash liquid, the more effective the person hygiene technique. TNTC means too numerous to count (a big number).]
Toilet Paper Only - 0.1 ml perineal rinse liquid number of bacteria :
TNTC (estimated total bacteria 30,000,000)
Toilet Paper and Peri-Bottle - 0.1 ml perineal rinse liquid Number of
Bacteria: TNTC (estimated total bacteria 10,000,000)
Bag-Type Sitz Bath Water Sample - 0.1 ml perineal rinse liquid number of bacteria : TNTC (estimated total bacteria 1,000,000)
Toilet Paper and Personal Hygiene Wipe - 0.1 ml perineal rinse liquid Number of Bacteria : TNTC (estimated total bacteria 24,000,000)
Hygenique only no Toilet Paper - 0.1 ml perineal rinse liquid number of bacteria : 112 (estimated total bacteria 112,000)
Hygenique Sitz bath Water Sample - Number of Bacteria : 0 (estimated total bacteria 0).[83]

3 key areas where toilet paper can cause you harm:
1. Toxic additives (manufacturing process and final product)
2. Bleaching with chlorine
3. Recycled paper containing bisphenols (BPA & BPS)

The following toxins are related to TP production (I am sure there are more if only I could find them. Getting any information on toxicity was very difficult):
Dioxin(dioxane) and BPA: Covered in their own sections. See below.

PEGs: This was a problem with flushable wipes. Many of them contained a variety of PEG compounds. Ethoxylated ingredients (like PEGs) on their own are of low concern to humans, however, the process of ethoxylation can leave behind trace amounts of carcinogens: ethylene oxide and 1,4-dioxane.[217]

A minority of people are allergic to Polyethylene glycol (a PEG). Allergy to a PEG is usually discovered after a person has been diagnosed with an allergy to an increasing number of seemingly unrelated products, including processed foods, cosmetics, drugs, and other substances that contain PEG or were manufactured with PEG. The amount of intake of PEGS has significant effects on clinical outcomes of affected patients.[2]

Undisclosed fragrances: There is no way to know what components are in these fragrances; we have no way to know if the ingredients are harmful or can cause an allergic reaction. Synthetic musks and phthalates are typically part of this undisclosed "fragrance". Phthalates are potent endocrine disrupting chemicals linked to obesity, hyperactivity in children and degraded sperm quality.[217]

Paraffin wax: This is made from petroleum by-products and can be absorbed into the skin. It may also be contaminated with carcinogens.[217]

Air Pollutants: The production of virgin wood pulp uses almost twice as much water as producing tissue from recycled materials and generates twice as many hazardous air pollutants. These air pollutants, such as formaldehyde and acrolein, can lead to respiratory problems; eye, nose, and throat irritation; and possibly cancer. Creating tissue from virgin pulp also generates 40 percent more sulfur dioxide, which can cause respiratory problems and acid rain, and releases thousands of times more particulates, which contribute to smog.[225]

Formaldehyde: Toilet paper has also been suspect in chronic irritation of the vulva. In a 2010 study, they found that toilet paper may be the blame for chronic irritation of the vulva because formaldehyde was found present to improve the strength of the toilet paper. Formaldehyde is a known carcinogen.[217]

Bleached Toilet Paper

What ever happened to "brown" unbleached toilet paper? It was quite popular in the 1970s, I was a happy buyer but somehow it disappeared. Virgin fiber or recycled, it is all white, why? We have been trained to trust only the purest white TP for our brown excremental stains, our poop. The environmental cost over the years (and growing unabated) has been huge, and unsustainable.

Bleaching is the process by which toilet paper is whitened [in my opinion completely unnecessary]. Most companies do this process because they say unbleached products are typically harsher to the touch. Aside from the waste, the process of bleaching toilet paper white leads to the creation of cancer-causing chemicals like dioxins and furans. Dioxins are extremely toxic and can enter by way of the air, waterways, soil, and the food chain. Exposure to even low levels of dioxins has been linked to hormone alterations (endocrine disruptors), immune system impairments, reduced fertility, birth defects, and other reproductive problems. Dioxins can be a carcinogen. The best course of action is to forgo chlorine entirely when bleaching.[217]

Trace concentrations of (dioxin) have been measured in some samples of bleached pulp and in some products manufactured from bleached pulp. In one study seven of nine bleached pulp samples were found to contain TCDD (dioxin) at levels ranging up to 51 parts per trillion. Eight of nine bleached pulp samples had TCDF (dioxin) levels ranging up to 330 ppt. [no quantities, conclusions or summary available!][65] Dioxins are bad for you at any amount.

Recycled Toilet Paper

A study published last month in the journal Environmental Science & Technology found widespread occurrence of BPA in paper products, including 80 of the 99 toilet-paper-containing samples tested. The researchers cited contamination during the recycling process as the source. This backs up findings from a previous study at the Wessex Institute of Technology that tracked estrogen pollution in wastewater to BPA in toilet paper.[67]

If you're set on a BPA-free toilet paper, then at least try a tree-free one made from sugarcane bagasse. Or a bidet. Even reusable toilet paper (though admittedly not for the faint of heart). Anything, please, but flushing a 300-year-old tree down the toilet.[67]

Seventh Generation – is an outstanding eco-friendly product line, no added fragrances or dyes, and will not irritate sensitive skin. Recycled fibers are not as absorbent as pure virgin fiber toilet paper brands, but Seventh Generation has accomplished an excellent 2-ply bath tissue that is made from 100% recycled paper with a minimum 50% post-consumer recycled paper. Seventh Generation 2-ply toilet paper is whitened without chemicals containing chlorine.[53]

The pulp and paper industry is among the world's largest generators of toxic air and water pollutants and waste products... Harmful chemicals like dioxin or phosphorus are some of the byproducts from the production process. For recycled toilet paper, less virgin wood fibers are needed, but research shows that recycled paper products are associated with 10-100 times higher concentrations of toxic chemicals such as BPA.[66]

According to Kimberly-Clark's 2005 Sustainability Report, the company used 3,113,000 metric tons of virgin fiber in 2005, an increase from the 3,067,000 metric tons of virgin fiber used in 2004 [this was the last time they publicly reported this tonnage in their sustainability report – I wonder why??]. Even assuming K-C is only meeting 14% of worldwide pulp need with pulp from the Canadian Boreal, this amounts to over 435,820 metric tons of Boreal pulp used by Kimberly-Clark in a single year. This has a disastrous impact on this ancient boreal forest, a 10,000-year-old ecosystem. For products that the company could be making from recycled paper.[266]

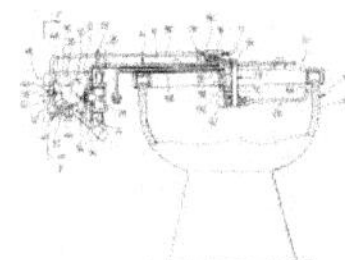

Dioxins

The process of bleaching toilet paper white leads to the creation of cancer-causing chemicals, such as dioxins and furans, which not only enter the air but also waterways, soil, and the food chain.[46]

"Dioxin," is the most toxic member of a class of related chemicals. It brings about a chain of events leading to various responses including: enzyme induction, immunotoxicity, reproductive and endocrine effects, developmental toxicity, chloracne, tumor promotion, etc. Some of these responses appear to be linear at low doses. Immunotoxicity and effects on the reproductive system appear to be among the most sensitive responses. [EPA][63]

According to the U.S. EPA's Toxics Release Inventory (TRI), pulp and paper ranks fourth among U.S. manufacturing industries in the release of dioxin and dioxin-like compounds to the air, and third in releases of these chemicals to water (U.S. EPA 2006d).[60]

When we buy toilet paper bleached with chlorine, we support pulp and paper mills that pollute our environment with dioxin and other toxic organochlorines. (Unbleached TP does not create dioxins.) It's true dioxin has recently been reduced 94% in US TP production, still no lower limit of safety exists for dioxins.[60] Dioxins can cause reproductive and developmental problems, damage to the immune system, interference with hormones and also cancer.[66]

The lion's share of environmental impacts from producing bleached kraft pulp comes from the bleaching process itself. [IMO totally unnecessary for "getting the job done"]. The choice of bleaching process is a major factor in a mill's environmental performance. In the USA, in order to meet Environmental Protection Agency rules, most paper is now 'elemental chlorine free' (ECF), which has led to a 94% reduction in dioxins, however the EPA's own rules state that there is no safe level of dioxin. Dioxin is known to cause reproductive problems, including low sperm counts and endometriosis and is implicated in a range of other health problems including diabetes, hyperactivity, allergies, immune and endocrine system problems.[60]

Dioxins are a group of highly toxic chemical compounds that are harmful to health. They can cause problems with reproduction, development, and the immune system. They can also disrupt hormones and lead to cancer. Known as persistent environmental pollutants (POPs), dioxins can remain in the environment for many years. They are everywhere around us. Dioxins are highly poisonous chemicals that are everywhere in the environment. Dioxins can stay in the body for a long time. They are stable chemicals, which means they do not break down. Once in the body, it may take between 7 and 11 years for a dioxin's toxicity to fall to half its original level.[72]

Since dioxin and related chemicals are so lipophilic (attracted to fat), they are mobilized from the adipose tissue during lactation and are eliminated through the milk. Therefore, nursing infants can have daily exposures 10 to 20 times higher than the background population. Subsistence fishermen also have elevated exposure due to the presence of these compounds in fish.[63] [US EPA 1994]

Dioxins cause a spectrum of morphological and functional developmental deficits. Fetotoxicity, thymic atrophy, and structural malformations are often noted. Delayed genitourinary tract effects have been observed, and recent studies reported behavioral effects. Highly exposed human offspring have exhibited developmental problems as well. Recently, hormonal and neurological abnormalities have been reported in infants from the general population. The complex alteration of multiple endocrine systems is likely associated with the spectrum of adverse developmental effects caused by dioxin and related compounds.[64]

BPA (bisphenol A)

Hold onto your hats, tree huggers, because you're not going to like what I'm about to say: BPA has largely been detected in recycled toilet paper.[67]

While recycled paper is, of course, a better option for the planet, here is another dirty little secret – bisphenols. Bisphenols like BPA and BPS have been discovered hiding inside recycled toilet paper. This is because thermal receipt paper, which is contaminated with bisphenols, BPA & BPS, ends up getting mixed into recycled paper products like toilet paper when we throw it into the recycling box [that's us folks]. Bisphenols like BPA are endocrine disruptors and studies have linked them to reproductive problems, early puberty, low sperm count, and breast cancer among other maladies.[217]

Bisphenol A (BPA) is a high-production-volume chemical associated with a wide range of health outcomes in animal and human studies. BPA is used as a developer in thermal paper products, including cash register receipt paper; however, little is known about exposure of cashiers to BPA and alternative compounds in receipt paper. The results of one study claimed only a few cashiers had detectable levels of total BPA or BPS in serum, whereas BPSIP tended to be detected more frequently. The researcher's conclusion was that thermal receipt paper is a potential source of occupational exposure to BPA, BPS, and BPSIP.[307] To a lesser degree this applies to every one of us using recycled paper intimately.

Choosing recycled paper does not clear the dangers of toxic chemicals and POPs. Research shows that there can be 10 to 100 times more toxic metal residues in recycled toilet paper than toilet paper made from virgin pulp, which is caused by the ink on recycled paper that cannot be completely removed during the process of de-inking. An important chemical in ink is BPA, bisphenol A, which is linked to increased rates of metabolic disorders and cancer. BPA can be found in high concentrations in recycled paper products and thus also in recycled toilet paper. On top of that, BPA is another persistent organic pollutant (WHO, 2016).[66]

BPA is an endocrine disruptor; infants and young children are said to be especially sensitive to the effects of BPA. Researchers have suggested that this type of action can affect puberty and ovulation, and that it may lead to infertility. The authors add: "The detrimental effects on reproduction may be lifelong and trans-generational". Research has linked even low-dose BPA exposure to cardiovascular problems, including coronary artery heart disease, angina, heart attack, hypertension, and peripheral artery disease. There is evidence that low-level exposure to BPA could contribute to insulin resistance and therefore diabetes type 2. Scientists believe BPA, with its estrogen-like behavior, could increase the risk of breast, prostate, and other cancers in people who were exposed to it in the womb. A systematic review published in 2016 found that exposure to BPA before birth increased the risk of wheezing and asthma.[72]

A study published last month in the journal Environmental Science & Technology found widespread occurrence of BPA in paper products, including 80 of the 99 toilet-paper-containing samples tested. The researchers cited contamination during the recycling process as the source. This backs up findings from a previous study at the Wessex Institute of Technology that tracked estrogen pollution in wastewater to BPA in toilet paper. Other carcinogenic chemicals like dioxin are being released into the atmosphere when conventional toilet paper is bleached. **Anything, please, but flushing a 300-year-old tree down the toilet.**[67]

The bottom line is that these days, there's no such thing as completely non-toxic toilet paper [not so, see Seventh Generation TP above] The recycled stuff is tainted with micrograms of BPA from other sources we also come into contact with, daily. But production of conventional tissue is a greater contributor to a toxic environment. For my money, the choice is in a bidet.[67]

Krikeys! Is that what the low boy is for? First, I thought it might be a dedicated baby bath. So I washed my infant son in it for awhile but he outgrew it after a year or two. Then I thought it was a training toilet, the seat area was too large and so LDP kept falling in. Besides, at that point, he was so used to taking a bath in it that the wanted to get naked and jump in.[12]

For example, a bidet is used for body washing [and occasionally babies] and requires much less water than a bathtub or shower. We calculated that a home equipped with a bidet would use, on the average, four gallons a day less than a home with no bidet due to less frequent use of the tub or shower. Likewise, a urinal requires about half the water of a toilet for each flush, so that during a day an average of five gallons might be saved.[91]

The amount of water we use to flush away our excrement is unimaginably staggering. It seems, in fact, that accurate figures are impossible because they are so high and so unpredictable. Some people have the habit of flushing the toilet before they use it, in dread of the possibility that the water standing in the pot just might have a stray pathogen in it, or a wee drop of piss, which they view with more alarm than radon in their walls. Low-flush toilets now in use compound the difficulty of adding up the numbers. Low-flush toilets are good news, but often people will flush them twice in order to make sure all the feces disappear. The feces phobia of Americans can be observed no more obviously than when watching the way some people become so upset when the toilet doesn't flush everything away the first try.[270]

If it takes 37 gallons of water to produce one roll of TP. This adds up to almost 2,000 gallons of water polluted just to make toilet paper for one person's use each year. If there was a program for universal bidet use in the USA, we could save more than 3.6 billion gallons of water each and every day at the very least. Another way that bidets may use less water than toilets is that people who use a bidet tend to feel cleaner, and they require fewer showers and baths as a result. This also helps to conserve water and waste less of this precious resource.[87]

Commercial paper making requires 199 gallons of water to process every gallon of pulp.[53] The manufacture of paper generates significant quantities of wastewater; as high as 60 m3/ton of paper produced. The raw wastewaters from paper and board mills can be potentially very polluting. Indeed, a recent survey within the United Kingdom industry has found that their chemical oxygen demands can be as high as 11,000 mg/l.[233]

Expansion of tree cover may assure Chinese toilet tissue manufacturers a steady source of wood fiber to feed an industry hungry for global market conquest, but at a cost. The goal is tree coverage of about 42 percent of China's landmass. Those trees will demand a lot of water in a country where water issues are already troublesome. World Rainforest Movement asks, "How can a biodiverse tropical forest be equated with a monoculture alien tree plantation?" The monocultures created in eucalyptus plantations, for example, displace indigenous plant and animal life, require tremendous amounts of chemical pesticides and fertilizers, and soak up such huge quantities of water that they have been planted to drain swamps.[48]

Our family had become accustomed to the wet cleansing wipes which we learned was a hazard not only to our own waste lines, but to the city's sewer systems. We love these units and are very happy with the purchase. In Hawaii, they are so popular, the local Toto store was out of stock. [1]

This non-randomized study recruited 221 ambulatory adults with anal diseases including eczema. Prior to the study, 55% of these patients (n = 120) used dry toilet paper to clean themselves after defecation. Of these patients, 60% who changed from dry toilet paper to water (bidet) after defecation had improved itching and burning symptoms; this was compared with 32% who changed from wipes to water, 30% who changed from dry toilet paper to wipes and 9% who changed from water to wipes. The authors concluded that cleaning with water was most effective. Patients who changed from wipes to water had a statistically significantly greater improvement in symptoms than patients who changed from water to wipes.[237] [Water vs. dry toilet paper vs. wipes containing Euxyl K 400 and polyethylene glycol as preservatives]

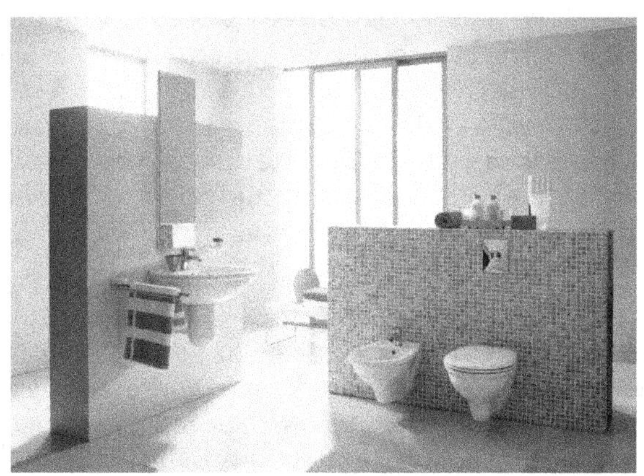

TP Ecology

Tissues, toilet paper, and other disposable products are responsible for unspeakable destruction of ancient forests around the world.[266]

With oil still choking the Gulf of Mexico, global climate change charging full-speed-ahead, and biodiversity shrinking by the week, the environmental consequences of toilet paper usage might seem a small concern. And yet, because everyone, everywhere poops, and because an ever-growing portion of the world's population uses toilet paper, and because much of that is virgin paper from ancient forests and tree plantations – this is an issue worth paying attention to, if for no other reason than the fact that toilet paper use has such a disproportionate impact on the environment. The production and use of toilet paper, from forest to flush, is yet another example of the complicated systems of resource use, manufacturing, and disposal that plague our planet caught between diminishing raw materials and a growing number of humans. Although it may not be as dramatic as the BP oil blowout, our daily toilet paper consumption raises something of an existential environmental dilemma: How can we meet this most basic of our needs without wrecking the planet? Or, in this case, how can we maintain our personal hygiene without destroying our virgin forests?[117]

The pulp and paper industry is one of the world's largest generators of toxic air and water pollutants and waste products. This industry is the world's largest user of fresh water and among the largest users of energy. And it destroys natural forests that are essential for clean air and water, the atmosphere's chemistry, wildlife habitat, indigenous cultures, spiritual inspiration and recreation. Instead of using trees harvested from biologically essential forest habitat, tissue paper products can be made from ecologically superior post-consumer recycled materials or agricultural waste.[71]

The pulp and paper industry has been criticized by environmental groups like the Natural Resources Defense Council for unsustainable deforestation and clear cutting of old-growth forest. The industry trend is to expand globally to countries like Russia, China and Indonesia with low wages and low environmental oversight. According to Greenpeace, farmers in Central America illegally rip up vast tracts of native forest for cattle and soybean production without any consequences, and companies who buy timber from private land owners contribute to massive deforestation of the Amazon Rainforest.[215]

In 2005 the Food and Agriculture Organization (FAO) of the United Nations, which monitors the state of the world's forests every few years, reported that 13 million hectares of global forests are lost annually, including 6 million hectares of what are described as primary forests-some of the most biologically diverse ecological systems in the world. And although ongoing depletion of forests in the Amazon is a focus of environmental alarm, a 2009 report published in Trends in Ecology and Evolution detailed the escalating threat to boreal forests in Russia, Alaska, Canada, and Scandinavia.[48]

According to the online magazine World Science, "the boreal, or northern forest, comprises about one-third of the world's forested area and one-third of the world's stored carbon." The U.S. and Canadian NGO ForestEthics reports that "Canada's boreal forest (alone) stores 23 percent of the planet's terrestrial carbon - more carbon per acre than any other ecosystem on earth, including tropical forests. However, Canada's old growth and intact forests are logged at a rate of five acres a minute, 24 hours a day".[48]

Monoculture plantations are increasingly incorporated in tree planting projects, such as those in China, and the paper industry often touts plantations as the solution to creating an ongoing supply of virgin pulp and fiber. The trouble is, a forest is far more than just a bunch of closely planted trees. Although the UN Food and Agriculture Organization considers plantations the environmental equivalent of native forest, the World Rainforest Movement asks, "How can a biodiverse tropical forest be equated with a monoculture alien tree plantation?" The monocultures created in eucalyptus plantations, for example, displace indigenous plant and animal life, require tremendous amounts of chemical pesticides and fertilizers, and soak up such huge quantities of water that they have been planted to drain swamps.[48]

The rainforests are important to our ecosystems. They produce the necessary oxygen that is vital for human survival, and each square mile contains thousands of unique species of animals. Every bit of extra toilet paper that we waste is contributing to damaging that fragile ecosystem.[187]

Old-growth and other ecologically important forests are being cleared to make tissue paper pulp. Many diverse natural forests, especially in the Canadian boreal, the Southeastern United States and throughout the developing world are being cleared, sometimes replaced by ecologically barren mono-culture plantations that are maintained with toxic chemicals, to produce tissue paper pulp. Thus, tissue paper products have an unacceptably high "footprint" on the planet. The world cannot afford another 100 years of business-as-usual in the paper industry.[71]

Recycling

We throw away enough paper to make toilet paper for a lifetime [Tim Spring, CEO of Marcal].[48]

[Creating fiber out of agricultural residue] Tissue pulp can also be made from non-wood alternative fibers, such as those from wheat straw and bamboo. Each year millions of tons of agricultural residue go to waste (2019).[225]

The case for recycling much or most of the paper that ends up in landfills - which can be made into perfectly acceptable toilet paper - is compelling, on several grounds. Various estimates place the quantity of waste paper tossed into U.S. dumps and landfills at 35-40 percent of total land filled mass. According to the University of Colorado's Environmental Center, "in this decade Americans will throw away over four and one-half million tons of office paper and nearly 10 million tons of newspaper...almost all of which could be recycled." Moreover, according to the Center, one ton of recycled paper (909 kilograms) saves 3,700 pounds (1,682 kilograms) of lumber and 24,000 gallons (90,849 liters) of water; uses 64 percent less energy and 50 percent less water to produce; creates 74 percent less air pollution; saves 17 trees; and creates five times more jobs than one ton of paper products from virgin wood pulp. So if recycling paper to make toilet tissue - the only paper product that cannot be recycled after use - makes so much sense, why is it not happening more often, in either U.S. or other global markets?[48]

Tim Spring, CEO of Marcal, a US company that has been making recycled toilet paper for more than 50 years – using nothing but recovered fiber –knows that customers are picky when it comes to soft tissue. He says he can deliver the desired softness using recycled materials. "Sixty percent of all paper manufactured ends up in landfills; only 40 percent is recaptured for further use," he says. "Most paper products can go through four cycles of recycling, with each cycle resulting in shorter fibers. Then various grades of recycled fiber can be blended in the toilet paper. **There is, Spring says, more than enough paper already out in the world to keep ourselves clean: "We throw away enough paper to make toilet paper for a lifetime".[117]**

LOL - OMG I can't believe you just post that. I felt like you were waking up the unspeakable - I think that talking about the bidet is almost a blasphemy in the world of bathroom fixtures. (lol) I never saw anybody so irreverent to this innocent piece of ceramic. I had a couple of good laughs - I have to admit ;) This is hysterical! I especially like the bidet as koi pond! Kathy [311]

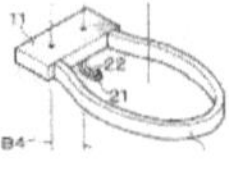

Marcal recycles office paper waste into toilet paper, "Using colored or printed recycled paper requires a de-inking process, which Spring describes as a soapy, watery bath for the ground-up magazines. "The water does the work, with the inks floating to the top of the tank, and clay residue sinking to the bottom. The top and bottom of the tank are skimmed," he says. "The water is recycled, too. It ends up as drinking water, which is cleaner than the local water sources. Nothing is lost, it is a closed cycle. The clay and ink residue is used as layering material in landfills or in road construction. So, in contrast to K-C, Spring concludes that producing recycled toilet tissue is the most logical response to consumer need for a one-time-use item: relying on local sources of recovered fiber, using less energy in manufacturing, cutting costs and fuel consumption, polluting less. The result is a desirable product for the marketplace and reusable byproducts as well.[48]

The case for recycling much or most of that waste paper - which can be made into perfectly acceptable toilet paper is compelling on several grounds. Various estimates place the quantity of waste paper tossed into U.S. dumps and landfills at 35-40 percent of total land filled mass. According to the University of Colorado's Environmental Center, one ton of recycled paper (909 kilograms) saves 3,700 pounds (1,682 kilograms) of lumber and 24,000 gallons (90,849 liters) of water; uses 64 percent less energy and 50 percent less water to produce; creates 74 percent less air pollution; saves 17 trees; and creates five times more jobs than one ton of paper products from virgin wood pulp.[48]

So if recycling paper to make toilet tissue - the only paper product that cannot be recycled after use - makes so much sense, why is it not happening more often, in either U.S. or other global markets? Looking at the corporation dominating the global toilet paper market provides some answers. According to Kimberly-Clark's 2007 Sustainability Report, North America ranks the lowest in use of recycled fiber, at about 20 percent for all K-C tissue products. By comparison, Europe's recycled-content tissue product use is about 36 percent and Latin America's is 67 percent.[48]

Only 2% of American households buy recycled-fiber toilet paper, compared to 20% in Europe.[66] If every US household replaced even one roll of virgin fiber toilet paper with one made from 100% recycled fibers, 423,900 trees would be saved.[46]

The logging that goes toward disposable paper products is especially frustrating given how much paper continues to be wasted. Each year, US consumers dump about 35 to 40 percent of all the paper they use into dumps and landfills. According to University of Colorado's Environmental Center, "in this decade Americans will throw away over 4.5 million tons of office paper and nearly 10 million tons of newspaper ... almost all of which could be recycled.[117]

A batch of paper can be recycled about 6 times. Most of the energy used to make virgin paper goes into pulping wood. Producing recycled paper uses 28-70% less energy and releases 95% less air pollution. Recycled paper is usually not re-bleached (or uses H_2O_2). Paper in landfills rots & releases CH_4 (greenhouse gas). One ton of recycled paper represents: 30,000 liters of water saved and 3,000 - 4,000 kWh electricity saved.[55]

We all can help quite painlessly; North Americans, who comprise only 7 percent of the world's population, consume nearly half of the world's tissue paper products. If every household in the United States replaced just one roll of 70-sheet virgin-fiber paper towels with 100 percent recycled towels, for example, they would save 544,000 trees - thousands of acres of forest land.[71]

[Bill Worrell, manager of the San Luis Obispo County Integrated Waste Management Authority in California] returned from a trip to Japan so impressed with the efficiency and superiority of the Washlet that he installed the system in the IWMA offices as a research model. Worrell discovered that consumption of paper products could be reduced by 50 to 90 percent. "This may not seem significant until we realize that Americans use more than 3.2 million tons of toilet paper annually, cutting down 54 million trees in the process," he says. "The production of each roll requires an average of 37 gallons [140 liters] of water. The average American uses 57 sheets of toilet paper per day, about 3.7 gallons of water per day figured for just for the manufacturing process. This compares to about 0.03 gallons [0.01 liter] per use of the Washlet".[48]

A Japanese company, Oriental Co. Ltd, won top prize at the Monozukuri Nippon awards, with the "White Goat," which turns 40 sheets of paper into one roll of toilet paper in 30 minutes! Here's how it works: When you feed the hungry machine 40 sheets of A4 office paper, the "White Goat" acts as a mini paper-recycling and processing factory. In 30 minutes the machine shreds and dissolves the waste paper into a liquid, spreads the liquid thin, dries it, and rolls it up neatly into toilet paper – without a tube in the middle. In a large business operation the "White Goat" can convert 1,800 shredded sheets into about 48 rolls of toilet paper in 24 hours. It uses between two and a half and four gallons of water per day to accomplish this feat. The final product is cheap: It costs a mere 11 cents per roll.[117]

Wipes and Fatbergs

Environmental groups have vocally condemned wet wipes for their plastic fibers, which, they say, add to the glut of garbage floating in the ocean and harm marine life.[68] As a result manufacturers have labeled some wet wipe brands as "flushable". Wet wipes, even "flushable" ones, when flushed down the toilet, have been known to clog internal plumbing, septic systems, & public sewer systems.[253]

The United States has largely ignored the bidet and its spin-offs, but it has warmly welcomed an alternative product: flushable wet wipes. These wipes became a cheapie work-around to address many of the same issues as the bidet, but they come at a much higher cost to the public. Wet wipes or wet naps were a mid-century invention used for everything from diaper changes to messy barbecue cookouts. In the medical literature there are cases of people found to be very allergic to the ingredients in moist toilet paper.[85,86]

A total of 6 women and 3 men with hand eczema were found to be allergic to (preservatives found in) different brands of moist towelettes used in diaper hygiene. Many were allergic to fragrance materials as well. The eruptions were mostly worse on the thumb and 2 adjacent fingers, with which the item was held. Five of the 9 were parents of infants, although no infant had a problem. Only 1 patient suspected the source.[88,86]

Q. Why is there discussion over moist wipes vs. toilet paper? A. The question of which TP is preferred helps me understand customer needs. It is common for users to try to save money but when it comes to this subject money is not the issue. The best TP may be only pennies more per application and is well worth the extra small cost. Adding high quality premium moist wipes into the equation is like having dessert.[69]

Fatbergs

City officials have reported that tens of thousands of moist wipes are recovered from the sewage system in New York City on a daily basis. The city officials have stated that these wipes do not break down like toilet paper, and they are costing taxpayers a considerable amount of money because they are clogging pipes and equipment and must be removed.[87]

So many people buy wipes for their convenience. Wet Wipes are relatively cheap to buy, but their disposal costs are immense and increasing daily. Wet Wipes have clogged innumerable home septic systems, often necessitating the expense of plumbers to clean up the mess. They've created major damage to sewer systems from Los Angeles to London. Once flushed, the wipes glom together with any fat from food waste and can form what are called "fatbergs"—iceberg-style blockages that can totally "stop up" a city's sewer system. To extract a fatberg and make the needed repairs can be incredibly pricey; in London back in 2015, one 10-ton fatberg cost the city $600,000. And last September, the city discovered another that's approximately 140 tons, which could very well cost 10 times as much to remove.[68,252-3]

"This unseen growing monster that lives in the sewers" Fatberg is important because it's something made by us, and that fascinates people. As a society, we've created this unseen growing monster that lives in the sewers, a place that we depend on but never see. It's also mysterious: it resides underground; and we don't know exactly what it's made of. For me, the fatberg is rather like the portrait of Dorian Gray: it shows our disgusting side. Just as in Oscar Wilde's novel, it is hidden away, getting worse and worse as we pile the accumulated sins of the city into it: cooking fat, condoms, needles, wet wipes, and of course human waste... The result can be quite liquid, or, like the Whitechapel fatberg, set like concrete... "Even small amounts of fatberg can kill" Is this a dangerous material to work with? Handled incorrectly, even small amounts of fatberg can kill... After my visit to Argent, I can tell you fatbergs absolutely reek. We can't let our visitors smell our fatberg samples – they could inhale particles of the fatberg itself. But hopefully, you'll never be so close to a fatberg again.[252]

Wipes build up with other waste, like congealed food fat, to form massive lumps called "fatbergs" that block entire municipal sewer systems. Now, imagine if you have a septic tank how these wipes will build up over time. Are you diligent about not putting left over cooking oil or bacon grease down the drain? The natural decay of waste inside your septic tank can't occur with these "indigestible" wipes and fat sitting in your tank.[128]

Family Cloths □A Cleaner Alternative

A bear and a rabbit are pooping in the woods. The bear asks the rabbit, "Do you ever have problems with poop sticking to your fur?" The rabbit finishes his poop and replies "No, I don't. Why?" "That's great!" says the bear as he grabs the rabbit by the ears, reaches between his legs and wipes.[298]

When our son was a baby we used a diaper service. We washed and re-used a lot of cloth diapers ourselves, but a diaper service was immensely helpful. My son would defecate in an impressive number of recycled diapers, we would toss them into the sealed bin they provided, then it would be picked up and clean diapers would replace them. Those diapers were recycled through countless babies and many many washings, and I have never heard of a problem with a diaper service. So why not family cloths? Perhaps there is room in the universe for commercial "family cloth" washing services, or a second income stream for diaper services?

There are alternatives to toilet paper even it you do not have a bidet. Some more eco-minded families have ditched the toilet paper altogether for rags instead. An entire cottage industry has sprouted up touting the sustainability of using "family cloths" instead of toilet paper. These are basically cloth rags you use, then store safely, rewash and keep using. You don't really need to purchase special ones. Cutting up old clothes and towels will suffice just fine.[217]

[Just go on the Internet and look for "Family cloth"]

Why would you use "family cloths?" Because they are cheap (free), biodegradable, and have no toxins in them (especially if you cut up old clothes). Below are comments from a dedicated "family cloth" user (via Buzzfeed online), whose name is withheld. This is good caution because there will be many people who are actually angered that someone would do this.

I personally have used the same washcloths for my butt drying for years now. Since I use a bidet those cloths rarely get visibly soiled, usually going into the laundry looking clean. We have established elsewhere in this book that bacteria will die on a relatively clean cloth – if they do not have moisture or sustenance.

"When people say, 'So, you just have piss rags laying around?' the answer is...yep. But not really. They stay corralled in a hamper for maybe a day at a time and then I empty them into the main hamper and then they're in the washing machine about twice a week. But my bathroom doesn't smell bad. It doesn't smell like a public toilet. It smells like my husband's beard balm".[265]

"A stain does not indicate filth. It's simply a discoloration caused when a substance containing intense pigmentation comes into contact with certain materials, like the natural fibers found in cloth. Modernity has coddled us into thinking that everything should be spotless and perfect, and, when marred, should be tossed and replaced. This mindset is part of what has gotten us into our current sad state of affairs, ecologically speaking. If my cloths get stained by menstrual blood and come out of the hot-water-with-bleach wash with reddish or brownish areas of discoloration, I honestly do not care and neither should you. We can all grow up and let go of our learned squeamishness for the sake of taking better care of our planet, our only home".[265]

[Editor's note: Some families definitely do use it for poop. One blogger who does writes, "I find it so much more comfortable and luxurious feeling. I feel cleaner. I also use it for 'that time of the month' which is extra-awesome. We ladies tend to feel icky in those days because it's tough to get totally clean with just paper. With a warm, wet cloth, I feel like I'm actually getting 100% clean. Full disclosure: sometimes I tag team it and use a bit of paper to wipe first, then a wet cloth for a more thorough clean." Another one advises using a spray bottle to clean your butt first before wiping with the cloth after doing #2 [basically a portable bidet].[265]

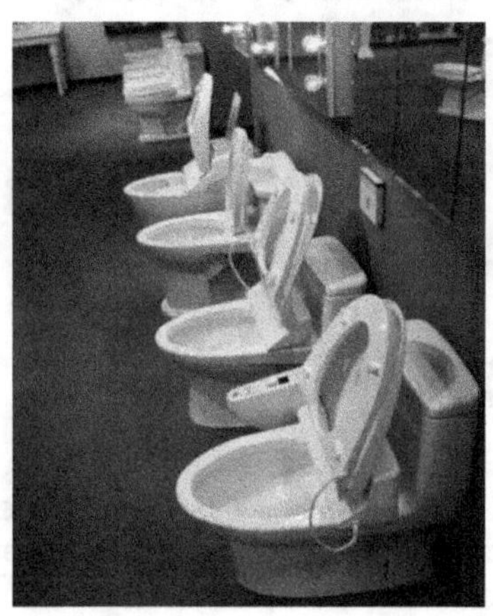

TP Sociology

(Toilet) culture is indeed a topic linked to a broad range of issues such as dirt and waste, cleanliness and hygiene, gender, sex and sexuality, embodiment and body excrements, human senses, social categories and divisions, spatial categorizations, socialization and communication, language and symbols, personal privacy, the politics of waste management, obscenity, violence and taboo, art and graffiti, just to mention a few.[204]

It is surprisingly hard to change habits learned at an early age, especially when it has been part of your culture for generations, if not time-out-of-mind. Particularly when the topic is effectively taboo in polite society.

Readers Please Note: I have worked very hard to portray how we process our wastes affects our own long-term survival, and the unsustainable ballooning costs of using toilet paper, and how bidets provide a very economical solution. Please do not take this personally, nor make it personal – I have my biases but believe that I have been an honest reporter on both sides of this story. Aside from some personal anecdotes about my use of a bidet, most words are straight quotes from peer-review research or industry reports. I have tried hard to be a good reporter of the facts despite the difficulties. Please respect this.

In my pre-adult years I was a toilet paper user, but now I have been a long-time user of a bidet. Researching and editing all of the peer-review research on all aspects of the bidet, has allowed me to see this social taboo from a different perspective, hopefully more independent of conventional thinking and prejudice.

I grew up in England in a house with no shower which was pretty typical I believe in the 1970s. We would fill the sink next to the bath and kneel over the bath using a beaker to wash our hair. It became quite an art form. In 1984, aged 11, I went on my first holiday abroad to Mallorca. Upon entering the hotel bathroom I excitedly exclaimed to my father that they had a special hair washing sink. I probably made the stinky egg face when he explained what it really was. I still washed my hair in it.[23]

State of the World

The toilet, I hold, is a rich and meaningful microcosm inasmuch as it provides clues for understanding the relationship between nature and culture, the perception of the human body and bodily waste in a given society, the collective representations.[204]

I think the subject of toilet is as important if not more so than other social challenges like literacy, poverty, education and employment. Rather the subject of toilet is more important because lack of excremental hygiene is a national health hazard while in other problems the implications are relatively closer to only those who suffer from unemployment, illiteracy and poverty.[7]

The enchanting features present the short-term benefits (of a flush-toilet municipal system), while hiding the slow, subtle, and surreptitious violence of market dependency, poor health, natural environmental degradation, and the polarities of abject and modernized poverty.... Flush-toilets are metabolized into society, as much as they are built into habits and values of people—often creating dependency, discomfort, and fear when these services change or fail. This level of dependency has not only led to wide spread atrophy in the colon, but also in people's imaginations as the fear of stool and hygienic obsession diminishes their ability to act. The atrophy of imagination and stultifying the desire for social and ecological harmony in daily practices is arguably the most structurally violent effect of flush-toilets.[234]

This all culminated with 19th and 20th century "Sanitation Revolution" age in which governments started enforcing strict hygiene rules, with organized garbage collection, development of public health departments, water treatment networks and more.[53]

Besides flush-toilets relatively unquestioned social integration, it is their complexity as an infrasystem that is comprised of a series of social and physical components that are regulated by public, private, and possibly informal institutions as a means to create, maintain, and improve a sanitation infrastructural service. Flush-toilets are one component or interface within a sanitation system necessitating to some degree a series of sewer mains, feeder pipes, pumps, different pressure systems, and drainage along with a series of different water and waste treatment systems.[234]

Body cleansing, like all universal and habitual activities, is subject to ritual uses and to a variety of philosophical and psychological meanings. Ritual cleansing is a practice that can be found in some form among all people and in almost all periods of history and still survives in many of the world's religions. Thus, circumcision, the washing of the hands at communion, washing of the feet, bathing in the holy Ganges, and other practices are all body-hygiene practices that have more symbolic than hygienic value. Most commonly purifying rituals such as these are performed after coming into contact with ritually contaminating things.[8]

A great many Europeans, for example, are repelled by the standard American bathroom in which the toilet and washing facilities are all together in the same space, as contrasted to European custom where the toilet is generally in a separate room - evidence of the clear difference in attitude toward bathing activities versus elimination activities. As some observers have argued, this is not so much a reflection on European problems with elimination as it is on the general American preoccupation with compulsive "cleanliness," devoid of any enjoyment, which results in our minimal "functional" bathrooms. The Europeans and the Japanese at least enjoy bathing, which presumably is more than many Americans do. In many parts of the world bathing is viewed and practiced as a shared, pleasurable activity - a scarcely possible feat in the average American five-by-seven foot bathroom, even if this desire was present.[8]

The anxiety and discomfort felt about excrement, combined with their attraction and fascination, represent a crucial anthropological paradox: the curious cultural taming of what appears to us as wild and uncontrolled. Like violence, cruelty, sex, abdominal desires and disobedient bodies, dirt seems to escape from the order that culture imposes; seems to... but does not... We should not underestimate the disciplinary power that culture produces. The dirt of human excrement is a useful topic to demonstrate that cultural ambiguity. Feces are indeed an intriguing matière à penser, which, however, has been amazingly neglected by anthropologists. Elsewhere I have attempted to explain that negligence. One reason, I believe, is that anthropologists in the field have been unable to rid themselves of their cultural codes of propriety. Home-based discomfort and rules of etiquette have prevented them from entering the dark world of defecation.[112]

A Normalized Habit

For most people in western countries, using toilet paper is a highly normalized practice which is often performed without being fully consciously aware of the practice itself or the consequences of using it. Cleaning after the use of sanitation, which includes using toilet paper for a lot of people, is a phenomenon of human behavior which is often associated with hygiene. Hygienic behavior is often motivated by the desire to avoid or remove things that are found to be disgusting. Using a bidet for example, removes the part of the toileting sequence where the user has almost direct physical contact between his/her hands and the feces he/she tries to remove. Most people value their health and the environment and yet persist in behaving in ways that undermine it.[66]

Toilet paper is a consumable necessity, but did you know that paper towels, a product mostly used out of habit, are some of the most overused and environmentally damaging paper products used today?[242]

When considering everyday habits and practices with a harmful environmental impact, toilet paper use would not be the first activity to come to mind. The use of toilet paper in Western countries is a very common habit and in most sanitation environments the only option of cleaning after using the toilet.[66]

Cleaning yourself after using sanitation seems to be a part of common human behavior. The problem is that some cleaning practices, like using toilet paper, have more harmful environmental consequences than other forms of cleaning, like using a bidet or a waterbrush.[66]

In the current form, individuals performing the practice of defecation have the meaning of cleanliness when using toilet paper, due to it having the least contact with feces. By using more advanced methods as the bidet or bidet sprayer, this contact with feces can be avoided in total. This would mean that water based methods would be the most clean option. As stated before however, such information targeting the conscious mind, does not make it likely that individuals change their behavior... People respond much more reluctantly when it comes to actually changing their behavior in ways that reduce their ecological footprint. Although people seem to care about their environment and personal health and hygiene, changing the habit of using toilet paper will probably not come with easy compliance.[66]

Old Attitudes, Other Attitudes

"What am I seeing oh! God, It is night soil, What a wonderful substance it is. It is excreted by the greatest of all Kings, Its odour speaks of majesty" French poet Piron in 'Royal Nightsoil', and as a result ostracised by the academic community.[7,114]

There was lot of jest and humor in medieval France relating to toilet habits and toilet appurtenances. Ballets were performed with basket of night soil in the form of hood, on the head or a tin plate commode moving around with toilet sounds. The clothes were spotted with accessories from the toilet. The actors were Etronice (night soil) Sultan Prime of Foirince (i.e. diarrhoea) etc.[7]

A lady of noble birth requested a young man to hold her hand. The young man suddenly feels the urge to urinate. Forgetting that he is holding the hand of a lady of noble birth, he relieves himself. At the end he says "excuse me Madam, there was lot of urine in my body and was causing great inconvenience".[7]

Over the ages human beings have employed various methods of personal cleansing following urination and defecation, including leaves, rags, seaweed, straw, grass, snow, sand, corncobs, coconut shells, newspapers, and catalog pages. Those with means enjoyed relative comfort and luxury: French royalty used lace, while hemp served upper class needs in many cultures and rosewater-infused wool was prized in ancient Rome. Defecating in running bodies of water was considered an efficient method of washing, and disposing of waste.[48]

The ancient Romans were economical about their use of their own waste. Human urine and feces were used in daily life in at least six different (and sometimes dubious) ways: Roman authors like Catullus attest to people using both human and animal urine as a mouth rinse that helped whiten their teeth; Columella wrote that old human urine was particularly useful for growing pomegranates, making them juicier and tastier; The ammonia in urine was also used to clean togas in a place called a fullery; various veterinary purposes such as sick bees could also be given human urine, and bird flu was cured by putting tepid urine on their beaks; The Romans frequently employed urine, dog feces, and sometimes human feces in tanning leather; also known as "night soil," the Romans used human feces and urine in their gardens.[292]

My 9 year old grand daughter and I saw one on a house tour. It's they only place in the back woods where you can see this sort of thing. We thought we would die laughing at how you switch from the toilet to the bidet without dripping all over the floor [classic bidet], and how do you wipe? With a towel? I have never laughed so hard in my life. My granddaughter and I still laugh about it, we just have to say the word "bidet" and we go nuts with laughter. It doesn't take much to make us happy with laughter here in the back woods. Am still laughing. Thank you who ever invented this, I have had so much happy time just discussing it.[12]

In ancient Osaka (Japan), money for night soil from shared toilets became a standard part of the landlord's income, and rent was based on the number of tenants—if someone moved out from a tenement house, the rent would rise, as the landlord would have less product to sell. Feces belonged to the house owner, while urine was the property of the tenants. Indeed, so large a part did night soil comprise of landlords' incomes, that the saying emerged, "the landlord's child is brought up on dung".[273]

A popular children's program on Dutch television in the 1970s and 1980s 'Ome Willem' always ended with a song containing the line 'Lus je ook een broodje poep?' (Would you like a poo sandwich?) It was the moment at which the children always loudly expressed their disgust... Conversely, several animals are fond of human excrements. There are countless stories about dogs and pigs that serve as sanitary agents in various societies. During my fieldwork in Southern Cameroon I had to protect my little daughter against the eager and impatient pigs while she was defecating in the bush. Among the Turkana people in Kenya mothers let dogs lick the buttocks of their babies after defecation.[112]

Gene Logsdon ponders why we have this fear of feces. He notes that some claim that our revulsion may have come naturally to protect us against diseases and conditions that can result from contact with our bodily wastes. Gene points out that parasite eggs and worms are found in feces and can then proliferate in nature, yet we do not fear them in this respect. He also points out that alcohol or smoke or automobiles do not invoke fear in us, even though they are as dangerous as occasionally touching shit. He concludes that fear of feces is mostly paranoia, just like our fear of spiders or snakes.[270]

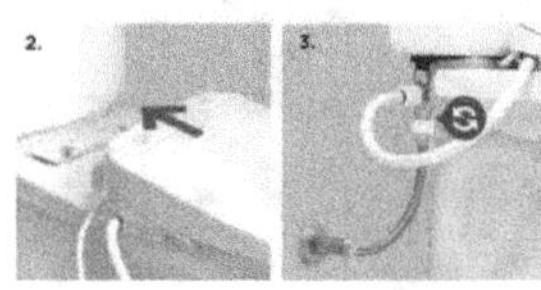

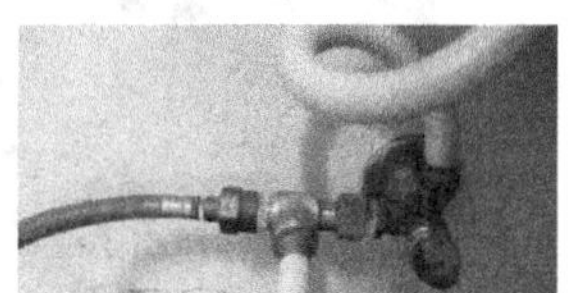

Not to ruin your dinner, but some people take a sip or two of their urine regularly to maintain health. I am not advocating anything of the kind, but the practice is ancient. Urine is, after all, not a particularly noxious liquid, but rather antiseptic, especially, I am told, as a skin lotion. Some of its champions claim it to be a blood purifier, whatever that means. Those well versed in the subject claim the only potentially harmful ingredient in urine is urea, which is present in such low amounts that urine is probably no more risky than whiskey, all things considered... There are many instances of humans eating feces too, although the practice is generally considered harmful. Even if it is not harmful per se, there are parasites and disease-causing bacteria to consider. I suppose the manure from a perfectly healthy human would not be harmful if ingested. Health officials say they find E. coli bacteria on restaurant tables as well as restaurant toilet lids and yet the human race survives while frequenting restaurants more than ever in history.[270]

Many other animals regularly eat poop, their own and that of other animals, including humans. Dogs, chickens, and hogs seem especially fond of human feces. There's an old bit of folk medicine in these part that calls for feeding rabbit manure to hens to make them lay more eggs. Mixing dried poultry manure back into livestock feed rations has been a practice for years. There are problems with this practice, for sure, but cattlemen have leaned to avoid most of them by feeding the stuff only in moderation. Once, at a livestock meeting years ago when this idea was first being discussed, I asked an animal nutritionist what he thought the public reactions might be to feeding manure. "Just don't tell them," he quipped. That, by the way, is when I started to distrust the agribusiness industry.[270]

I certainly don't want to sound as if I am advocating using excrement for food, but nevertheless the long history of doing so may have the good effect of shocking all of us into a less fearful attitude toward our bodily wastes. We take into our mouths the most delectable and fragrant foods, but as they make their extremely intimate way through our bodies, we assimilate some of the "good" nutrients in them and what's left turns into what we consider repulsive corruption. Some of what we assimilate may be more corrupting to our bodies than what we eliminate, but anyway, the very second that our excrement exits our bodies we wouldn't touch it with a vaulting pole. As I said earlier and will probably say again, if shit were white and smelled like roses, our problems with waste management would be over.[270]

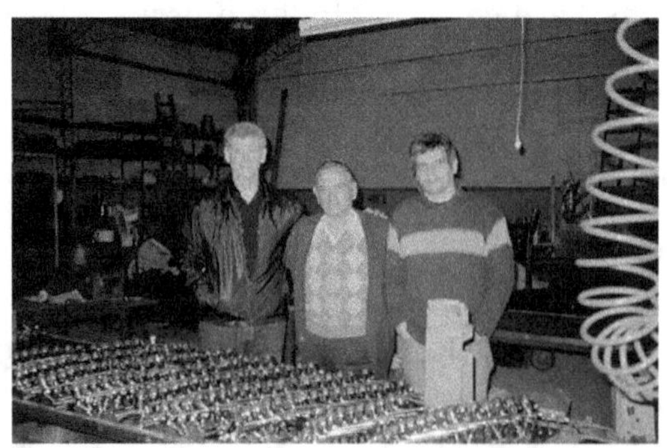

Two Hundred Years Of Habit

Despite often being overlooked, in most parts of the world a day without tissue paper products is unthinkable.[251]

If stranded on a desert island with only one "necessity", what would you choose? 49% chose toilet paper as their greatest island necessity (ahead of food!).[119]

The more deeply one delves into cleanliness behavior, the more apparent it becomes that our primary concern is with visual rather than actual cleanliness. Dirt and soiling exist only in the eyes of the beholder. The most compelling evidence is to be found in perineal hygiene, where even the most apparently elegant and fastidious are often to be found wearing under drawers soaked in urine and smeared with fecal matter.[295]

The concept of dirt offers people the opportunity to order their life. The old functionalistic view that order is the heart of culture has never been abandoned, however loudly the structural-functionalist tradition may have been criticized. The classification of dirt shows how that order is constituted and where the boundaries between good and bad, right and wrong, inside and outside lie. Mary Douglas's concept of 'matter out of place' has been most influential here. Excretions of the body comprise the most strongly felt 'matter out of place' and therefore the most informative pointers of cultural boundaries.[112]

We should not underestimate the disciplinary power that culture produces... It would be a mistake to disregard the qualities of the substance itself: color, texture, moisture, and smell. Feces do seem to have a 'natural' dirtiness. The fact that they are almost universally regarded as disgusting supports this view. Still, we need to keep in mind that 'natural' reactions in the strict sense of the term do not exist in human societies. Children acquire culture by being taught the dirtiness of their feces. Their initial attraction to feces suggests that 'natural aversion' is doubtful. The working of the senses is largely formatted by cultural lessons... However, bringing them up in conversation – or writing, as I am now doing – makes them dirty because we feel that they should not be discussed in public. Shit is an intimate product. We part with it in private and there it should remain. By talking and writing about it, it becomes a matter out of place; it disturbs the order of proper behaviour.[267]

"We don't want to know where our shit goes," says Larry Robinson, a Sebastopol City Council member and practicing psychoanalyst. "Every organism's waste is another organism's food, but there's some notion that we as human beings are above the cycle of life and death. We don't want to know what comes out the other end".... A scholar of European history, Robinson traces our break with nature back to the plagues of the Middle Ages and the industrial revolution that followed. By the 19th century, our modern system of enclosed, underground sewers was in place, just in time for Scott Paper's introduction of the first toilet-paper roll in 1890. Since then, there's been no looking back. Our break, Robinson postulates, has metastasized into an abject terror of sexuality and defecation. "Our ethos of conquest and environmental destruction has distracted us from nature and our own bodies," he says.[6]

Human defecation is considered at least in poor taste by many and obscene by others, and whatever attitudes one holds are apt to be pursued with vehemence, if not vengeance... All manner of verbal and social conventions are attempted to disguise or mitigate our activities, such as running water to mask the sound of other running water. While such stratagems are more or less successful, they all ultimately fail with respect to telltale odors - a source of considerable concern and embarrassment for many.[8]

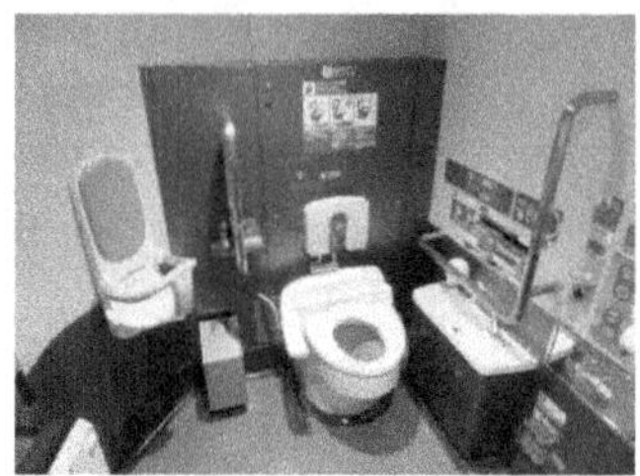

We Know, But☐

"My contribution deals with another kind of institutionalized not knowing: not knowing about defecation. That not knowing does not refer to lack of knowledge on the part of informants about their defecation practice. They know very perfectly well, to the smallest detail, when, where, and how they defecate... The classification of dirt shows how that order is constituted and where the boundaries between good and bad, right and wrong, inside and outside lie. Mary Douglas's concept of "matter out of place" has been most influential here... Excretions of the body are the most strongly felt matters out of place and, therefore, the most informative pointers of cultural boundaries".[112]

When I am in public and have to take a crap (which is very rare, but happens) I use another method, while still sitting on the toilet, I flush it about 3 or 4 times to make sure water in bowl is clean, reach hand into the water, scoop some up and repeatedly scrub my anus, and flushing every couple times. After anus feels squeaky clean, I dry off with a wad of tp, pull up pants, and go over to sink and wash hands thoroughly. I don't like to have to resort to that, but I absolutely have to feel clean about myself, and that's the only way I can do it in public restrooms. Wiping off with a wet paper towel isn't good enough for me. Nothing worse to me than the feeling of walking around with shit stuck to my ass, N O C A N D O ! ![12]

In order to assess the dirtiness of feces we do have to pay attention to its in- or out-of-place character. Questions such as 'what,' 'where,' 'whose,' and 'how it is present' are relevant. 'Whose,' as we know, can make a lot of difference: whether it is my own or someone else's? My child's or my neighbor's? Does it come from a human being or from an animal? From what kind of animal? Experiences of disgust may vary enormously, depending on the answers to the above questions. 'How it is present' refers to whether feces are present physically or only in the text we read, the conversation we have, the film we watch.[112]

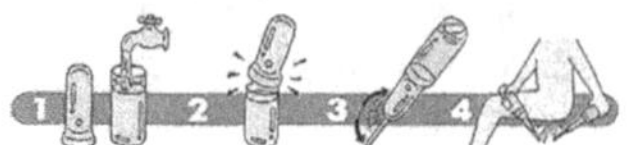

Our fear of feces is so great that even in very respectable journals and books, you will find protectors of the public health insisting that every last speck of feces be eliminated from any possible contact with human activity or our very lives are in danger. This is cultural thinking, not scientific thinking. Not commonsense thinking either. Well-intentioned literature emphasizes that a gram of feces may contain a million bacteria, and woe to us. But so might a gram of good humus. A gram of feces may contain billions of viruses, but again, that dos not mean that these viruses all cause human disease. If a person is healthy, so is his manure. Some "parasites" in manure are actually parasites of other possibly harmful bacteria. Nor is the problem of parasite worm eggs avoided simply by flushing feces down the toilet: worm eggs can survive for awhile even in wastewater treatment plants. Their effort to do so is leading us in a quite the opposite direction... Technically the high temperatures of typical garden composting will kill all pathogens in human manure in a very short time.[270]

"Perhaps most famously, Sigmund Freud argued that at this age, the child is going through an "anal stage" when he or she gets immense psychosexual pleasure from the development of anal control through toilet training. Research in children shows that the subject of the humor changes as they develop. In very young children, a game of peek-a-boo is the subject of much amusement. In the preschool years, we see a fascination with jokes about excrement and toilets... The three-year-old running round the house saying "poo" or pretending to go to the toilet is arguably appreciating the incongruity of being able to use the word liberally. They are also playing with the action of toileting, the social conventions around it and the possible shameful consequences of incontinence. Toilet humor is therefore a natural part of their development... So, for parents whose toddlers find excrement very funny, it is probably a sign of healthy development if they are also learning to use the potty in an appropriate way. It shows they are thinking about and reflecting on what they are learning, and upon the social rules that surround it. And for parents to be able to have a little laugh with their toddler about this learning process, shows them that it is an okay subject for discourse. This limits the shame and embarrassment that occurs during the inevitable accidents."[278]

My feces in my body are in the right place as long as they do not stay there for too long and do not worry me. My feces may become dirty if someone starts to draw special attention to their presence and tries to discredit my human body as 'a sack of shit.' My feces are thus removed from their orderly place in the universe and put directly in our collective faces by talking about them. Neither do feces in the lavatory disgust us as long as they are our own.[112]

So I just came to Korea recently and there's a few budget Japanese toilets kicking around but I'll be honest with ya here I don't know what the fuck I'm doing and hitting buttons on the control panel these bad toys feels like a good way to get absolutely sloshed. Any pointers on why there are seventeen options on Japanese toilets and which one to go with?[84]

Basically, the huge industry of producing toilet paper could be eliminated through the use of bidets.[20]

Industry Feeds the Obsession

First of all, what happened to unbleached natural colored TP? Sometime in the 1970s or so it simply disappeared as a available product. What is the connection between incredible whiteness and then smearing it with smelly, generally dark stained feces? What is with the obsession over softness, I mean it is way overboard. We know the TP manufacturers can recycle softness if they are motivated. Why is water cleansing so unnerving for some, when it is used to clean your anus? In my researches on the web, a strong minority of our nation (at least) are addicted to TP. Look at the pics of empty TP shelves during the coronovirus.

Although some form of paper has been used for perineal wiping purposes for centuries, it wasn't until 1857 that an American inventor named Joseph Gayetty announced the arrival of the first purposefully-made toilet paper advertised as: "Gayetty's Medicated Paper for the Water-Closet." Gayetty took aim at his greatest competitors, the newspapers, magazines and catalogs that people were already using in their toileting practices. And, in the truest of American traditions, he used "scare tactics" to warn potential customers of the chemicals (including toxic arsenic) in these alternatives, in order to win over new buyers.[258]

In my opinion, the international paper industry is still using "scare tactics" to get us to buy increasingly chemicalized TP. This is an interesting reversal from the first days of TP. Back then the scare was getting chemicals on your butt by not using TP, the scare today should be that there are so many chemicals in TP that it is safer not to use it.

Of course, humanity has not always depended on long, silky tree fibers (logged from ancient forests or massive monoculture tree plantations, transported hundreds or thousands of miles, bleached with harsh chemicals, air-dried with high-octane machines, and then shipped thousands more miles again) for personal cleansing.[117]

There Is A Better Way

Sim Van der Ryn (author of **The Toilet Papers**) cites a 1974 report that Los Angeles at that time was dumping about 235 million gallons of primary treated effluent and 100 million gallons of secondary effluent into the ocean every day. "It got me to thinking, " he writes, "the nutrients in all that effluent, much of it from flush toilets, if converted to fertilizer, would be the equivalent of 200 tons of 7-14-12 fertilizer... Each ton when applied to soil would provide the nutrients to grow 25 tons of vegetables. Thus each day, L.A.'s waste provides the nutrients to grow 5000 tons of vegetables, enough to provide everyone in Los Angeles with a pound or two of fresh produce daily.[270]

The Bill Gates Foundation sponsored a toilet fair to inspire innovation for redesigning the concept of the toilet... University of Colorado Boulder scientists were awarded a $780,000 grant to fund the building of a waterless and solar powered toilet. The toilet uses concentrated sunlight to sanitize and breakdown the toilet waste to make biological charcoal, also known as "biochar." The biochar can then be used as a fertilizer for farming, offering farmers a natural alternative to chemical fertilizers. The foundation expects to be able to test its first prototypes within the next three years.[69]

All I'm asking for is that we all try to keep an open mind on the subject. Prohibiting the use of biosolids on farmland does not solve the problem facing us. If this material is toxic to the food chain, burying it in a landfill is only a temporary solution. How many centuries can we continue to do that? Or as an alternative, how long can be afford to flush it into the atmosphere by burning it? I'm suggesting that despite the formidable problems involved, we should keep open minds on the possibilities of using biosolids for fertilizer. We know how to keep biosolids safe, but we can't utilize this knowledge until we figure out a way to keep people from throwing potentially toxic substances into the toilet, and, so far, we lack the will to confront the problem. But we can have both our flush toilets (or at least some fluids toileting) and our fertilizer. Perhaps we all can at least agree that applying biosolids to non-food-producing lands represents an ecologically appropriate solution to an enormous waste disposal problem.[270]

I bought a bidet 3 months ago and haven't pooped anywhere else since...until today. I saw someone on Reddit say that it changed their life, and only $20 on Amazon. So I gave in and bought one. BEST. PURCHASE. EVER. I absolutely LOATH LOATHE using any other toilet. It's that awesome... Seriously! After a recent trip to Indonesia, where every toilet has a butt squirter, we came to the realization that it makes so much more sense than using tons of paper. We installed one as soon as we got home. Our friends are all skeptical and think it's a bit gross but we always tell them, if you got poop on your arms, would you wipe it with paper or wash it off?[226]

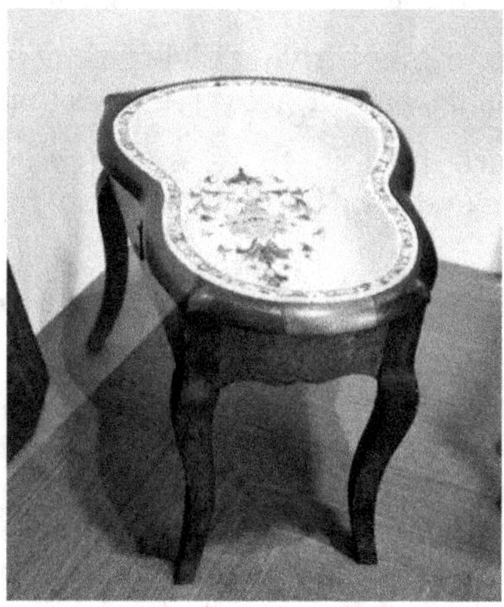

ca 1880 - Rolled and perforated tissue paper as we're familiar with today was invented. Faced with the consumers' resistance toward the "unmentionable" product. Scott Company was too embarrassed to put their name on their product, as the concept of toilet paper was a sensitive subject at the time, so they customized it for their customers... hence the Waldorf Hotel became a big name in toilet paper.[220]

A History Of Elimination

This section comprises a timeline history of how we have taken care of our human waste. It is a fascinating interweaving of the development and use of sanitation systems, toilet, bidet, wash water, and toilet paper from diverse industry and academic sources.

Building a timeline from scratch would have been a huge undertaking in itself. I am indebted to two commercial sources that have provided a good chunk of the information presented in this timeline: Toilet Paper World website, "Toilet Paper History" (www.toiletpaperhistory.net/); and History on the Porta-Potty website (www.portapotty.net/ plumbing/). Both of these companies do excellent work in their particular line of business. If you are interested they have a lot more history than I selected in this timeline. I encourage y'all to visit these websites.

6000 BC - Examples of early "plumbing" could be seen in 6000 B.C. Mesopotamia, where slaves hand-carried large pots of water up from the river.[122]

4000-3000 BC - The first copper water pipes were discovered by archaeologists in the Indus River Valley of India.[122]

3000 BC - The oldest archeological discovery of working toilets dates back to Scotland. In their Neolithic settlement Skara Brae scientists found remnants of the stone huts, fully equipped with drains that extended from the recesses in the walls. This extremely early and very sophisticated example of toilet technology was not seen in in other more advanced cultures for thousands of years, managing even to remain superior to any design in the entire world.[53]

Egyptian ruler Menes supports a thriving civilization spanning over 3000 years by constructing canals, basins, and irrigation ditches to hold floodwater.[122]

2750 BC - At Mohenjo-daro in India, there are privies with seats connected to a highly developed drainage system where waste water from each house flows into the main drain.[7]

2700 BC - Water pipes are crafted from clay and chopped straw in the Indus River Valley in India.[122]

2500 BC - Egyptians were credited with developing their own copper pipes to construct elaborate indoor bathrooms in pyramids. Egyptians used this same ingenuity to build detailed irrigation and sewage systems for public use.[122]   In Mohenjo-Daro, there existed highly developed drainage system where waste water from each house flowed into the main drain.[7]   Lothal (near Ahmedabad in Western India) the people had water borne toilets in each house which was linked with drains covered with burnt clay bricks. To facilitate operations and maintenance, it had man-hole covers, chambers etc. It was the finest form of sanitary engineering.[7]

2100 BC - Innovative Egyptians fashion group sitting toilets out of stone. Toilets are also built in tombs as the Egyptians believe the dead should be provided with everyday necessities in the afterlife.[7,122]

1500 BC - Complex sewage disposal systems with rudimentary flushing toilets are credited to King Minos of Crete.[122]

1000 BC - A flush type toilet was discovered on Bahrein Island in the Persian Gulf,.[7]

500 BC - Lead-lined bathtubs began to appear in northern Greece.[122]

Ancient Greece - Chamber pots are in use and urine is collected to bleach sheets.[115]

Ancient Rome - All public toilets have a stick with a sponge attached to its end that soaks in a bucket of brine so citizens can have a tool to freshen up with.[53]

50 BC - The Chinese first made paper with short lengths of bamboo and then later added cotton linen rags which were soaked in water and pounded into swollen pulp. This was then formed into sheets and dried.[53]

52 AD - Rome boasts an estimated 220 miles of aqueducts, water channels, and pipes used to supply public wells, baths, and homes.[122]

70 AD - There is a considerable Roman trade in urine, which is collected in pots on street corners and used for stiffening and dyeing cloth. The Emperor Vespasian (AD 69--79) imposes an unpopular tax on the use of public urinals, which becomes known as Vespasiani.[292]

105 AD - Ts'ai Lun, a Chinese court official, has his name linked to the invention of paper. Most likely, Ts'ai mixed mulberry bark, hemp, and rags with water, mashed it into pulp, pressed out the liquid, and hung the thin mat to dry in the sun.[53]

200 AD - the first papermaking process was developed in China.[53]

500-600 AD - The first documented use of actual toilet paper was in sixth century China, with the scholar Yan Zhitui writing, "Paper on which there are quotations or commentaries from the Five Classics or the names of sages, I dare not use for toilet purposes".[119]

500-1000 AD - Early Middle Ages - Sexual excesses and the increase of sexually transmitted diseases lead to the elimination of the public baths.[116]

ca. 700 - Arabs were known to make writing paper and were the first to use linen in the process.[53]

700-1500 - Considered the "dark ages of plumbing and hygiene," where disease, cesspools, and human excrement abound.[122]

851 AD - during the Tang Dynasty (618 - 907 AD), an Arab traveling through China wrote about the Chinese people, "They do not wash themselves with water when they have done their necessities, but they only wipe themselves with paper.[47] Islamic tradition prescribes that you should wipe with stones or clods of earth, rinse with water, and finally dry with linen cloth. Pious men actually carry clods of earth in their turbans and carry small pitchers of water solely for this purpose. These men traditionally blot the end of their penis with pebbles or clods of earth.

Others blot against a wall, which gave rise to a practical joke among the non-Muslims living around the Eastern Mediterranean – they dusted the outdoor walls at penis level with good old ground hot pepper. Ouch![120]

ca. 1300 - According to the OED, the word privy is 600 years old, and means a private place of ease, a latrine, a necessary; hence privy house and privy stool.[18]

1391 - Toilet paper was officially introduced in China, when big sheets of paper were produced in Korea for the Chinese royal family for personal hygiene uses. The area now known as the Zhejiang province annually manufactured ten million packages of between 1,000 and 10,000 sheets of perfumed toilet paper.[119]

1519 - The provincial government of Normandy in France made provision of toilets compulsory in each house.[7]

1596 - The flushing toilet was invented by Sir John Harrington, who was a British nobleman and godson to Queen Elizabeth I. He invented a valve that when pulled would release the water from the water closet and suggested flushing at least twice a day. (Rumor has it that this is where the name the "John" originated.)[122]

1668 - Edict issued by Police Commissioner Paris, for construction of Toilets in all houses.[7]

1690 - William Rittenhouse and William Bradford of Germantown, PA built the first North American papermaking mill at Wissahickon Creek, near Philadelphia. They used rags as the raw material. Rags were boiled, rinsed, and beaten to a pulp, then pressed to get the water out and dried to become paper.[53]

1700 - Initially, colonial Americans used corncobs and leaves to cleanse where toilet tissue is used today. Then, when newspapers became available they were used. Also, the Sears catalog and the Farmers almanac were later used. The Almanac had a hole in it so it could be hung on a nail or string.[53]

1700s - The cleaning of the body becomes very important in Europe.[116] European urbanites in the 18th century deposited waste in chamber pots and threw sewage into city streets.[122]

1710 - The bidet appears to be an invention of French furniture makers in the late 17th or early 18th century, although no exact date or inventor is known.[16]

1716 - Hemp was first used in an experiment as a raw material for paper making in Europe.[53]

1718 - First reference to paper as toilet paper.[53]

1726 - The earliest written reference to the bidet.[16]

1750 - A manual pump handle allowing for upward spraying was installed, and thus bidet á seringue, or bidet with syringe, came into the lives of avid bum cleaners everywhere.[274]

1775 - The first US paper money. Stephen Crane sells currency-type paper to engraver Paul Revere, who prints the American Colonies' first paper money. Revere's transaction is on display in the Crane Museum.[53] Alexander Cummings secures the first patent for the flushing toilet.[122]

1800s - Connections between personal cleanliness and disease evolve in England during the century, particularly after the formation of germ theory in the 1880s.[118]

1810 - The English Regency shower is introduced, where water is plumbed through a nozzle and sprayed onto the shoulders. Water runoff is collected and reused as it is pumped through the shower again.[122]   The US census reported 179 paper mills in 17 states with an output of 3,000 tons. But the supply of rags was not sufficient to fuel the growth and demand for paper. European imports of rags became very expensive.[53]

1822 - A US tariff on rags was implemented to help the papermakers in the US. From here on, the industry grew steadily into its world dominance of today.[53]

1829 - The first hostelry in the world opens with indoor plumbing at the Tremont Hotel in Boston. Soon, soap used during bathing catches on for hygiene purposes.[122]

1833 - The White House is plumbed with running water on the first floor. Upstairs plumbing is introduced 20 years later when President Franklin Pierce is in office.[122]

1844 - Money Paper. Crane patented a method to embed silk threads into banknote paper to foil counterfeiters.[53]

1851 - The first public toilets were introduced in London's Crystal Palace.[122]

1854 - Wood pulp first successful used in US to make paper. Mechanical wood pulp or groundwood, as the new pulp was called, was used to supplement the supply of rags, and the mixture of rags and wood pulp produced a paper suitable for the times.[53]

1856 - Albert L. Jones, a New York City inventor, in 1871 was the first to use corrugated paper as a packing material for shipping kerosene-lamp chimneys and other glass. Goodbye sawdust and straw – over the next two decades cardboard evolved into today's familiar sandwich, corrugated stuffing between two layers of linerboard.[53]

1857 – Conventional toilet paper was finally introduced by Joseph C Gayetty. "Gayetty's Medicated Paper for the Water Closet" contained aloe and was marketed as a means to cure sores and prevent hemorrhoids.[119] Gayetty took aim at his greatest competitors, the newspapers, magazines and catalogs that people were already using in their toileting practices. And, in the truest of American traditions, he used "scare tactics" to warn potential customers of the chemicals (including toxic arsenic) in these alternatives, in order to win over new buyers.[258]

1860 - The importance of indoor running water is emphasized after Louis Pasteur publishes research on dangerous bacteria. Homes are built with large, immobile cast-iron sinks, inspiring the phrase "everything but the kitchen sink".[122]

ca 1880 - Rolled and perforated tissue paper as we're familiar with today was invented. Faced with the consumers' resistance toward the "unmentionable" product. Scott Company was too embarrassed to put their name on their product, as the concept of toilet paper was a sensitive subject at the time, so they customized it for their customers... hence the Waldorf Hotel became a big name in toilet paper.[220]

1880 - The first actual paper produced for freshening up is sold in England... The individual squares are sold in boxes, not rolls. This paper is very coarse - the type the British prefer today.[53]   Toilet curtains make their appearance.[7]

1883 - German inventor Carl Dahl discovered adding sodium sulfate to the caustic soda pulping process produced a very strong pulp. This was called the Kraft process; Kraft means strong in German.[53]

1885 - The first comprehensive sewer system in the US is built in Chicago. Homes still lack indoor baths; public bathing facilities charge five cents for adults and three cents for children.[122]

1889 - Sewage Treatment for the first time in the world.[7]

ca 1890 - In rural America, it was still common practice at the time to leave a corncob hanging from a string in the outhouse for people to wipe themselves with: Once the kernels were removed and the cob allowed to dry, the remaining kernel husk was fairly soft, or softer than a rock, at least. The string, meanwhile, indicated that the cob was, you guessed it, communal. By the late 19th century, the Sears catalog had become the toilet paper of record for many folk.[119]

1890 - Toilet Paper on a roll was introduced by the Scott Paper Company and quickly becomes the nation's leading producer of TP.[6,69]

ca 1900 - Modern plumbing allows the bidet to move from the bedroom to the bathroom.[16]   Mussel shells were still very popular in coastal regions prior to toilet paper's popularity.[120]

1907 - Soft, fluffy toilet paper introduced. The original American product is sort of like crepe paper.[120]

1907: Scott introduces Scott paper towels. The Sani-towels became the first disposable paper towel in America used in Philadelphia schools to help prevent the spread of common colds.[258]

1915 - American servicemen see the company name Thomas Crapper & Co. stamped on European toilets and later spread the common US term for toilet, "crapper," when they build American plumbing infrastructures in the 1920s.[122] Kimberly Clark begins producing absorbent cellulose wadding called Cellucotton. This was to be used as a bandage material in WW1. Subsequently army nurses begin adapting this material for menstrual use. Three years later this becomes Kleenex.[53]

1920 - Kimberly Clark forms the company Cellucotton Products to market Kotex sanitary napkins. The KC Company owners are afraid to associate with this 'unmentionable' product. Kotex is first advertised in 'Ladies home journal' in 1921 but the ad is restricted in explaining the products use.[53]

1923 - Plumbing and toilets in Japan were not widely used until after the Great Tokyo earthquake in 1923 when the importance of sanitation to reduce disease was realized.[184]

1930 - Northern Toilet Paper was marketed as "splinter-free," eventually leading to a softness arms race amongst toilet paper manufacturers as the presence of at least one roll of quilted cotton per restroom became expected by the general public.[119]   1930s - Use of the Sears catalog declined in the 1930's due to the fact that they started printing on glossy, clay-coated paper. Many people complained to Sears about this glossy paper.[120]

1931 - Scott makes ScotTowels, the first paper roll towel. They market using 'Mr. Thirsty Fibre" for absorbency, wet-strength and economy.[53]

ca 1940 - Albert Einstein was an honorary member of the Plumbers and Steamfitters Union.[122]

1942 - St. Andrew's Paper Mill in Great Britain introduces two-ply toilet paper. Before this toilet tissue was one-ply and not very soft.[53,120,220]

1946+ - After World War II, Western toilets became more widespread. Toto and other companies borrowed technology from France, the United States and Switzerland and, as the Japanese have done with other technologies, improved it and adapted it their own purpose.[184]

1955 - Scott advertises toilet tissue on TV for the first time.[53]

1957 - Hans Maurer invents the Clos-o-Mat combined Water Closet and bidet. He calls this device a "shower toilet".[24]

1964 - Toto imports a bidet-toilet called Wash Air Seat from American Bidet Co.[184]

1966 - Toto Ltd. of Japan introduces their first version of the bidet.[184]

1966 - Clos-O-Mat introduces "Junior," a toilet seat bidet, but abandons production after two years due to technical and performance problems.[24]

1968 - Kimberly Clark introduces disposable diapers named Kimbies. This became Huggies in 1978.[53]

1973 - The Great Toilet Paper Shortage occurs in 1973 after evening talk show host Johnny Carson makes a joke that there is an acute shortage of toilet paper in the United States. The next morning, 20 million viewers buy up all the toilet paper they can find. By noon that day, most stores are out of toilet paper. Scott Paper showed video of their plants in full production to the public and asked them to stay calm – there was no shortage. The video was of little help. The panic fed itself and continued. They finally got the shelves restocked three weeks later and the shortage was over. To date it is the only time in American history that the consumer actually created a major shortage.[69,120]   Charmin patented a process to make their paper softer through air-drying, fluffing up the paper in favor of the conventional method of squeezing it flat.[119]

1977 - Shipments of Western-style toilets overtook Asian-style ones for the first time.[184]

1980 - Toto Ltd. of Japan introduces Washlet, the first "paperless toilet", a toilet seat unit with warm-water bidet functions and a heated seat, which also dries the user after washing.[184]

1986 - The first sensor flushing toilet is introduced in Japan.[122]

1992 - Low-flow toilets are manufactured to conserve water, with both single and dual flush. Low-flow toilets consume 1.6 gallons per flush compared to 3.5 - 7 gallons per flush in older models.[122]

1999 - A paperless toilet is introduced in Japan. It is complete with a washing/rinsing mechanism, a blow-drying component and a heating element.[53]

2001 - Charmin purchased Moist Mates claiming to introduce the first pre-moistened bath tissue. They call it Charmin Fresh Mates.[53]

2003 - The manufacturing of squat style toilets ended in Japan.[184]

2005 - As of 2005 Toto has sold 20 million Washlets and sells about 3 million a year.[184]

2008 - Marcal Paper Products announces a new brand of eco-friendly and recycled paper products, Small Steps. All of the products in the line (toilet paper, paper towels, facial tissue, napkins, etc) are made from 100% recycled material and contain a high percentage of post-consumer recycled content.[53]

[Submitted by Francesco – Italy] - I can't believe on the year 2005 there's still people who don't EVEN KNOW what a bidet is and who are... SCARED of it! I read once that American people think they are the world's cleanest (not to mention, the world's most civilized)... well they're so clean and civilized, that they keep the most delicate parts of their body (not only the anus ok?) dirty!! Wow it's terrible! I don't even want to think about sex among dirty persons like them![12]

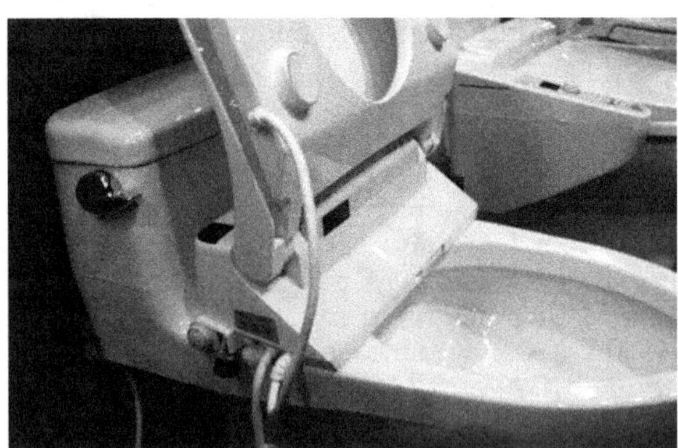

While I have used the USABIDET system for over ten years and to complete satisfaction, I did eventually need to "upgrade" to an ADA height toilet. I was pleased to learn that USABIDET had already anticipated this growing trend and now makes a longer supply line to compensate for the added height of an ADA toilet.[41]

References

1   https://www.amazon.com/TOTO-SW2034-01-Electronic-Elongated/dp/B00
UCIOWRM
#customerReviews
Amazon website-Toto Corp
Washlet website – Reviews

2 https://en.wikipedia.org/wiki/
Wikipedia is a free content encyclopedia, being written collaboratively by contributors from around the world. These topics have been used in this book.
Islamic hygienical jurisprudence
Kraft Process
Xylospongium
1880 US Census
Anal Fissure
Toilet Paper
Polyethylene glycol (PEG)
Etc.

3 https://www.usatoday.com/story/life/2019/01/18/bidet-popularity
-us-bathroom-toilet-tushy-kohler-american-standard/2590700002/
USA TODAY Jan. 18, 2019
Do you need a bidet? The butt-spritzing toilet gizmos are making a splash in the U.S. Carly Mallenbaum,

4 http://www.japaninc.net/mag/comp/2000/10/oct00 _blowfish.html
Japan Inc. website, Blowfish section

5 http://www.filipino.ca/bidet/testimonials.asp
Hyjet bidet website: Testimonials

6 http://www.metroactive.com/papers/sonoma/11.20.03/bidets-0347.html
North Bay Bohemian Magazine November 20-26, 2003
A Bidet Runs through It: How a simple stream of water can change one man's life
R. V. Scheide -- The North Bay Bohemian is a free weekly newspaper

7 http://www.sulabhtoiletmuseum.org/history-of-toilets/
History of Toilets exploring history of sanitation & hygiene
A paper presented at International Symposium on Public Toilets held in Hong Kong on May 25-27, 1995 -- Dr. Bindeswar Pathak, Ph.D., D.Litt.
Founder, Sulabh Movement and Sulabh International Museum of Toilets

8   (book) Viking/Compass, 1975
The Bathroom, Alexander Kira

9 https://goaskalice.columbia.edu/answered-questions/hey-whats-bidet
Go Ask Alice website, Columbia University Education: "Hey, What's a Bidet?"

10   http://www.showerbaby.net/testimonials2.html
Shower Baby website: Testimonials

11   Int Arch Occup Environ Health. 2010 Feb;83(2):123-32.

Cancer mortality in a Swedish cohort of pulp and paper mill workers.
Andersson E1, Persson B, Bryngelsson IL, Magnuson A, Westberg H.
Department of Occupational and Environmental Medicine, Sahlgrenska University Hospital, Göteborg, Sweden.

12   http://www.poopreport.com/Consumer/Content/Bidet/bidet.html,
The Bidet: Not Just for Hairy European Women Anymore
Colon Bowell. The Poop Report website Posted 9.7.02001

13   Personal communication from Neil Munro, principal at Clos-O-Mat UK

14 http://www.consumerreports.org/cro/toilet-paper.htm
Consumer Reports website - Toilet Paper

15   Some people use the terms like "toilet seat bidet" to describe these types of fixed-position bidets, and I use the acronym TSB to describe them throughout this book.

16   http://en.wikipedia.org/wiki/Bidet
Wikipedia on-line encyclopedia: Bidet

17 http://www.sanicare.com/
History of the Bidet -- Sanicare website sells many models of bidets

18   This definition is from the Oxford University Press Dictionary© supplied with Word Perfect 10, the word processing program I used to write the original edition of this book.

19 http://www.hygenique.com/
The Hygenique™ system website: Testimonials

20 https://www.scientificamerican.com/article/earth-talks-bidets/
Scientific American online: ENVIRONMENT (2019):
Dear Earth Talk Wipe or Wash? Do Bidets Save Forest and Water Resources?
EarthTalk is produced by E/The Environmental Magazine.

21 PRI's The World - Public Radio, Arts, Culture & Media June 03, 2014
"Why I don't like bidets, but Iove the washlet" -- Alina Simone

22 http://www.ertravel.com/erro/archive/2000/122.html
Comments from Er Travel's website:

23 https://www.bbc.com/news/magazine-28237337
BBC News Magazine, 15 July 2014: The imaginative ways readers use bidets

24 (book) "25 Years of Clos O Mat", 1983
Peter Maurer, Hans Maurer Closomat AG.

25 http://www.clos-o-mat.com
Clos-O-Mat website

26   Med Eng Phys. 1996 Sep;18(6):515-8
The development of the Port-a-Bidet - a portable bidet for people with minimal hand function
Burkitt J, etal -- Brunel Institute for Bioengineering, Brunel University, UK.

27   https://brightthemag.com/how-do-you-get-people-to-give-a-shit-about-shit-tell-poop-jokes-616627c6d4f8
How Do You Get People To Give A Shit About Shit? Tell Poop Jokes.
Sarah Bell, water systems lecturer at University College London
Bright Magazine website

28   https://biobidet.com/pages/why-you-should-use-it
Biobidet website: "Why you should use it" -- Biobidet is an online seller of bidets

29   Infect Control. 1986 Feb;7(2):59-63
Physiologic and microbiologic changes in skin related to frequent handwashing.
Larson E, Leyden JJ, McGinley KJ, Grove GL, Talbot GH.

30   Dermatology. 1997;195(3):258-62
Effects of soap and detergents on skin surface pH, stratum corneum hydration and fat content in infants
Gfatter R, Hackl P, Braun F.
Department of Pediatrics, University of Vienna, School of Medicine, Austria

31   Ostomy Wound Manage. 1998 Mar;44(3A Suppl):62S-69S; discussion 70S.
Soaps and detergents - understanding their composition and effect
Kirsner RS, Froelich CW. -- Department of Dermatology and Cutaneous Surgery, University of Miami School of Medicine

32   Dermatol Clin. 2000 Oct;18(4):561-75
Modern skin cleansers.   Ertel K.
Sharon Woods Technical Center, Procter and Gamble Company, Cincinnati, Ohio

33   Skin Therapy Lett. 2003 Mar;8(3):1-4.
Cutaneous cleansers.   Kuehl BL, Fyfe KS, Shear NH.
Department of Medicine, University of Toronto Medical School, Ontario, Canada

34   http://www.portable-bidet.com/testimonials.asp?page=2
Personal+Hygiene Systems website: Testimonials
Personal+Hygiene Systems in an online seller of bidets

35   http://www.thefactoryoutlet.com/bidets.htm
The Factory Outlet website: Bidet information
The Factory Outlet is an online seller of a number of bidet models

36   http://www.magicjohn.com
Magic John website - Main page information
Magic John is an online seller of bidets

37   Nurs Times 2002, April 2-8;98(14):56-9
Can tap water be used to irrigate wounds in A&E? -- O'Neill D.
A&E Department, Frimley Park Hospital, Camberley, Surrey

38 www.nytimes.com/2007/09/27/garden/27bidets.html?pagewanted=all&_r=1
Flush With Excitement: Pitching the Modern Bidet -- MARA ALTMAN
The New York Times, Home and Garden section, SEPT. 27, 2007

39   Dis Colon Rectum. 2005 Dec;48(12):2336-40.
Sitz bath: where is the evidence? Scientific basis of a common practice.

Tejirian T1, Abbas MA. -- Department of Surgery, Section of Colon and Rectal Surgery, Kaiser Permanente, Los Angeles, California

40   ANZ Journal of Surgery Volume 78, Issue 5 May 2008 Pages 398-401
WARM SITZ BATH DOES NOT REDUCE SYMPTOMS IN POSTHAEMORRHOIDECTOMY PERIOD: A RANDOMIZED, CONTROLLED STUDY -- Pravin J. Gupta

41   https://www.americanhygienics.com/blank-page
USA Bidet – testimonials -- USA Bidet is an online seller of bidets

42   J Gastrointest Surg. 2009 Jul;13(7):1274-8.
Comparison of clinical effects between warm water spray and sitz bath in post-hemorrhoidectomy period. -- Hsu KF1, Chia JS, Jao SW, etal
Division of Colon and Rectal Surgery, Department of Surgery, Tri-Service General Hospital, Taipei, Taiwan.

43   Zentralbl Hyg Umweltmed. 1998 Feb;200(5-6):562-70.
[Anal hygiene in perianal skin diseases--compatibility of water moist and dry toilet paper]. [Article in German] -- Brühl W1, Schmauz R.
Erstes Deutsches Darmzentrum, Vlotho-Exter.

44   Uttered by a proctologist I know when I told him about this book.
Proctology deals with anorectal problems.

45   https://www.urbandictionary.com/define.php?term=bidet
Urban Dictionary: Bidet (top definition) -- Anonymous March 12, 2005

46   http://articles.mercola.com/sites/articles/archive/2014/10/18/bidet-use. aspx
Dr. Joseph Mercola website -- Why Most Americans Don't Own a Bidet

47   Ann Colorectal Res. 2017 March; 5(1):e46479
Water Stream in Bidet Toilet Commode as a Cause of Anterior Anal Fissure: A Case-Control Study -- Pankaj Garg,1,2, Pratiksha Singh2
Colorectal Surgery Division, Indus Super Specialty Hospital, Mohali, Punjab, India -- Garg Fistula Research Institute, Panchkula, Haryana, India

48   http://www.worldwatch.org/node/6403
World Watch Magazine, May/June 2010, Volume 23, No. 3
Flushing Forests -- Noelle Robbins
Worldwatch Institute, Vision For a Sustainable World

49   European Journal of Public Health, Volume 28, Issue suppl_4, 1 November 2018
Unpleasant side effects due to bidet toilet use -- L Catarsi G Troiano etal
Post Graduate School of Public Health, Department of Molecular and Developmental Medicine, University of Siena, Siena, Italy

50   https://www.refinery29.com/en-us/bidet-health-benefits-for-women
Bidets Are Trendy-But Are They Healthy? -- CORY STIEG
Refinery 29 website-AUGUST 3, 2018, 10:20 AM

51   American Journal of Obstetrics & Gynecology Supplement to JANUARY 2018
Bidet toilet use - the association with abnormal vaginal colonization and preterm birth in high risk pregnant women, a prospective study -- Yoomin Kim
Samsung medical center, Seoul, Korea, Republic of Korea

52   Obstet Gynecol. 2013 Jun;121(6):1187-94.
Effect of bidet toilet use on preterm birth and vaginal flora in pregnant women.
Asakura K1, Nakano M, Yamada M, Takahashi K, Sueoka K, Omae K.
Department of Preventive Medicine and Public Health, Keio University School of
Medicine, Shinjuku-ku, Tokyo, Japan.

53   http://www.toiletpaperhistory.net/
http://www.toiletpaperhistory.net/toilet-paper-facts/toilet-paper-fun-facts/
Toilet Paper History -- Toilet Paper World website

54   http://www.epa.gov/grtlakes/seahome/housewaste/src/paper.htm
Paper Facts: "Recycling paper uses 60% less energy than manufacturing paper
from virgin timber." -- EPA website

55   http://budker.berkeley.edu/PhysicsH190_2012/Hosseinzadeh%
20Recycling_Energy_Conservation.pdf
Energy and Environmental Considerations in Recycling, 11 April 2012
Griffin Hosseinzadeh -- Physics H190

56   www.theguardian.com/environment/2009/feb/26/toilet-roll-america
American taste for soft toilet roll 'worse than driving Hummers': Extra-soft,
quilted and multi-ply toilet roll made from virgin wood causes more damage than
gas-guzzlers, fast food or McMansions, say campaigners
Suzanne Goldenberg -- US environment correspondent
The Guardian newspaper website 26 Feb 2009

57   http://www.nlm.nih.gov/medlineplus/ency/article/000862.htm
US National Library of Medicine Encyclopedia -- Balanitis

58   http://thegreentoilet.blogspot.com/2008/02/so-why-is-toilet-paper-white-
anyway.html
Making your bathroom eco-friendly. Quick tips for restaurant & store owners,
homeowners, apartment dwellers, and more!
The Green Toilet website

59   Preventive Medicine Reports Volume 6, June 2017, Pages 121-125
Bidet toilet use and incidence of hemorrhoids or urogenital infections - A one-
year follow-up web survey
TeppeiKiuchia, Keiko Asakurab, Makiko Nakanoa, Kazuyuki Omaea
Department of Preventive Medicine and Public Health, School of Medicine, Keio
University, Tokyo, Japan

60   http://environmentalpaper.org/wp-content/uploads/2017/08/state-of-the-
paper- industry-2007-full.pdf
The State of the Paper Industry: Monitoring the Indicators of Environmental
Performance
Susan Kinsella, Gerard Gleason, Victoria Mills, etal
Steering Committee of the Environmental Paper Network

61 xxx

62   Journal of Obstetrics and Gynaecology Research 30 September 2010
Habitual use of warm water cleaning toilets is related to the aggravation of
vaginal microflora

Mitsuharu Ogino, Koichi Iino, Shigeki Minoura
Department of Obstetrics and Gynecology, Toyama Hospital, International Medical Center of Japan

63   Environ Health Perspect 102(Suppl 9)157-167(1994)
The Mechanism of Dioxin Toxicity - Relationship to Risk Assessment
Linda S. Birnbaum
U.S. Environmental Protection Agency, Health Effects Research Laboratory, Research Triangle Park, NC

64   Toxicology Letters Volumes 82–83, December 1995, Pages 743-750
Developmental effects of dioxins and related endocrine disrupting chemicals
S Birnbaum
Experimental Toxicology Division, National Health and Environmental Effects Research Laboratory, United States Environmental Protection Agency, Research Triangle Park, NC

65   Environ. Sci. Technol. 1989, 23, 6, 643-644
Assessing potential health risks of dioxin in paper products
Russell E Keenan, Michael J Sullivan
ChemRisk, Portland OR
[no quantities, conclusions or summary provided!]

66   University of Utrecht: An interdisciplinary research on the alteration of the environmentally harmful human activities revolving around the use of toilet paper -- Wiping the Habit
Willemijn Jüttner, Environmental Social Sciences and Environmental Policy
Rens van Dijke, Innovation Sciences
Chris Dekker. Cognitive and Neurobiological Psychology

67   https:www.huffingtonpost.com/jennifer-grayson/eco-etiquette-is-my-toile_b_1008317.html
Eco Etiquette: Is My Toilet Paper Toxic?
Jennifer Grayson -- Huffington Post website

68   https://www.theatlantic.com/technology/archive/2018/03/the-bidets- revival /555770/
The Bidet's Revival -- MARIA TERESA HART
The Atlantic Magazine website MAR 18, 2018

69   http://blog.toiletpaperworld.com/
"Flushable Wipes vs. Toilet Paper: What Works Best?
Toilet Paper World Blog, including Toilet Paper Encyclopedia

70   www.nrdc.org. Retrieved 19 February 2016
Paper Industry Laying Waste to North American Forests
Natural Resources Defense Council website

71   www.laondaverde.org/media/pressreleases/041118a.asp
FLUSHING FORESTS DOWN THE TOILET
Allen Hershkowitz -- Natural Resources Defense Council

72   https://www.medicalnewstoday.com/articles/221205.php
How does bisphenol A affect health?

Christian Nordqvist -- Reviewed by Suzanne Falck, MD, FACP
Medical News Today Website Thu 25 May 2017

73   http://www.pri.org/stories/2014-06-03/why-i-dont-bidets-iove-washlet
Why I don't like bidets, but love the washlet
Alina Simone
Public Radio International's "The World", June 03, 2014

74   Dis Colon Rectum. 2002 Mar;45(3):370-6.
 The perineorectal reflex The perineorectal reflex in health and obstructed
defecation.
Gosselink MJ, Schouten WR.
Department of Surgery, Erasmus Medical Center, Rotterdam, The Netherlands.

75   Gastroenterologist. 1998 Jun;6(2):96-103
The technical aspects of biofeedback therapy for defecation disorders
Rao SS
Department of Medicine, University of Iowa College of Medicine, Iowa City

76   Am J Gastroenterol. 1988 Aug;83(8):827-31
Studies of manometric abnormalities of the rectoanal region during defecation in
constipated and soiling children: modification through biofeedback therapy
Keren S, Wagner Y, Heldenberg D, Golan M.
Institute of Gastroenterology, Hillel Jaffe Memorial Hospital, Hadera, Israel

77   Dig Dis Sci. 1987 Aug;32(8):841-5
Bowel habits in young adults not seeking health care.
Sandler RS, Drossman DA.

78   J Am Geriatr Soc. 1989 May;37(5):423-9.
Constipation in the elderly living at home. Definition, prevalence, and
relationship to lifestyle and health status.
Whitehead WE, Drinkwater D, Cheskin LJ, Heller BR, Schuster MM.
Johns Hopkins University School of Medicine, Baltimore, Maryland

79   http://www.holistic-online.com/ Yoga/hol_yoga_breathing_traditional.htm
#Low
Everything you want to learn about yoga and more.
Dr. J. Mathew - Chief Editor and Webmaster
HolisticOnLine Yoga Supersite

80   (book) "A Voyage to the Levant" 1741
Joseph Pitton de Tournefort

81   http://www.sandman.com/Intimst.html#Why
IntiMist Electronic Bidet web page
Sandman Telecom & Bidet Experts website

82   Popular Science August 22, 2002
How long do microbes like bacteria and viruses live on surfaces in the home at
normal room temperatures?
Edited by Bob Sillery, Research by Reed Albergotti and Emily Bergeron

83   http://hygenique.com/hospitals.html
Hygenique website: For Hospitals

84 https://www.reddit.com/r/Frugal/ a_month_ago_i_bought_a_bidet_for_25 /in_that_time
Reddit website: r/Frugal

85   Dermatology. 1995;191(4):299-304
Tolerance to different toilet paper preparations: toxicological and allergological aspects -- Blecher P, Korting HC
Department of Dermatology, Ludwig Maximilian University, Munich, Germany.

86   Ned Tijdschr Geneeskd. 1991 Jun 8;135(23):1048-9
[Peri-anal allergic contact eczema with dyshidrotic eczema of the hands due to the use of Kathon CG moist toilet wipes - Article in Dutch]
de Groot AC, van Ulsen J, Weyland JW.

87   https://www.bidet.org/blogs/news
(1) Baby Wipes Versus Bidets: Moist Wipes are Not the Solution According to City Officials in New York
(2) How much water does a bidet really use?
Bidet.org website (commercial)

88   Am J Contact Dermat. 2001 Dec;12(4):189-92.
Baby-wipe dermatitis: Preservative-induced hand eczema in parents and persons using moist towelettes.
Guin JD, Kincannon J, Church FL.
Department of Dermatology, Univ of Arkansas Medical Sciences, Little Rock AR

89   https://blog.studentsville.it/top-10-tips/everyday-life/say-okay-to-the-bidet-your-10-questions-answered/
Studentsville Blog - Say Okay to The Bidet: Your 10 Questions Answered
Whitney Richelle   1/31/2017
http://www.linkedin.com/in/whitneyrichelleschaefer

90   https://thoughtsfromparis.com/stories/came-glorious-glorious-bidet/
Thoughts From Paris blog: How I Came to Own a Glorious, Glorious Bidet
D. J. -- an American in Paris

91   UTILITY RATINGS AND 0-1 PROGRAMMING IN HOUSING DESIGN 8.4
Richard Hobson and Imre Kohn
The Pennsylvania State University

92   Acad Emerg Med. 1998 Nov;5(11):1076-80.
Wound irrigation with tap water
Moscati RM, Reardon RF, Lerner EB, Mayrose J.
Department of Emergency Medicine, State University of New York at Buffalo

93   Eur J Surg. 1992 Jun-Jul;158(6-7):347-50
Comparison between sterile saline and tap water for the cleaning of acute traumatic soft tissue wounds.
Angeras MH, Brandberg A, Falk A, Seeman T.
Department of Surgery, Medical Microbiology, University of Goteborg, Ostra, Sweden.

94   J Accid Emerg Med. 1997 May;14(3):165-6
Tap water as a wound cleansing agent in accident and emergency.

Riyat MS, Quinton DN.
Department of Accident and Emergency, Leicester Royal Infirmary NHS Trust.

95   Acad Emerg Med. 1998 Nov;5(11):1076-80.
Wound irrigation with tap water
Moscati RM, Reardon RF, Lerner EB, Mayrose J.
Department of Emergency Medicine, State University of New York at Buffalo

96   Plast Surg Nurs. 1989 Fall;9(3):117-9.
Water Piks: wound cleansing alternative.
Trelstad A, Osmundson D.

97   J Clin Periodontol. 2000 Feb;27(2):134-43.
Clinical benefits of oral irrigation for periodontitis are related to reduction of pro-inflammatory cytokine levels and plaque.
Cutler CW, Stanford TW, Abraham C, Cederberg RA, Boardman TJ, Ross C.
Baylor College of Dentistry-TAMUS, Dallas, Texas

98   Am J Public Health 1984; 74:479-484.
The Role of Skin Absorption as a Route of Exposure for Volatile Organic Compounds (VOCs) in Drinking Water
HALINA SZEJNWALD BROWN, PHD, DONNA R. BISHOP, MPH, etal
Office of Research and Standards, Massachusetts Department of Environmental Quality Engineering

99   J Water Health (2015) 14 (1): 68-80. Volume 14, Issue 1 February 2016
Bidet toilet seats with warm-water tanks - residual chlorine, microbial community, and structural analyses
Toru Iyo Keiko Asakura Makiko Nakano Mutsuko Yamada Kazuyuki Omae
Department of Health Sciences, School of Allied Health Sciences, Kitasato University, Kanagawa, Japan

100   J UOEH. 2014 Jun 1;36(2):135-9.
A survey on bacterial contamination of lavage water in electric warm-water lavage toilet seats and of the gluteal cleft after lavage.
Hideki KATANO1), Kumi YOKOYAMA2), Yasushi TAKEI3), etal
School of Health Sciences, Tokai University, Japan

101 Journal of Hospital Infection Vol 97, Iss 3, November 2017, Pages 296-300
Public health and healthcare-associated risk of electric, warm-water bidet toilets
A.KanayamaKatsuseaH.TakahashiaS.Yoshizawabc, etal
Department of Infection Control and Prevention, Toho University Faculty of Nursing, Tokyo, Japan

102   World J Gastrointest Oncol. 2016 Apr 15; 8(4): 402–409.
Colorectal cancers and chlorinated water
Ahmed Mahmoud El-Tawil
Department of Surgery, University Hospital Birmingham, Birmingham UK

103   J Water Health (2015) 14 (1): 68-80.
Bidet toilet seats with warm-water tanks - residual chlorine, microbial community, and structural analyses
Toru Iyo Keiko Asakura Makiko Nakano Mutsuko Yamada Kazuyuki Omae

104   Personal reminiscence
Geoff Wilcox
a personal friend and a frequent traveler and resident of India.

105   Surg Gynecol Obstet. 1975 Sep;141(3):357-62.
Wound cleansing by high pressure irrigation.
Rodeheaver GT, Pettry D, Thacker JG, Edgerton MT, Edlich RF.

106   Ann Surg. 1978 Feb;187(2):170-3
Evaluation of wound irrigation by pulsatile jet and conventional methods.
Brown LL, Shelton HT, Bornside GH, Cohn I Jr.

107   Burns. 2001 Jun;27(4):413-4
Perianal burn caused by using the bidet.
Shulman O, Wolf Y, Hauben DJ.

108   Contact Dermatitis. 1995 Feb;32(2):83-7
 Effects of water temperature on surfactant-induced skin irritation.
Berardesca E, Vignoli GP, Distante F, Brizzi P, Rabbiosi G.
Department of Dermatology, University of Pavia, IRCCS Policlinico Italy.

109   Contact Dermatitis. 2001 Sep;45(3):146-50.
Do cool water or physiologic saline compresses enhance resolution of experimentally-induced irritant contact dermatitis?
Levin CY, Maibach HI.
University of California at San Francisco Medical Center, San Francisco, CA USA.

110   Infect Control. 1986 Feb;7(2):59-63
Physiologic and microbiologic changes in skin related to frequent handwashing.
Larson E, Leyden JJ, McGinley KJ, Grove GL, Talbot GH.

111   https://www.buzzfeed.com/sarahburton/the-bidet-is-a-bido
I Cleaned My Ass With A Bidet And This Is What Happened: Not that I needed to, because girls don't poop or anything.
Sarah Burton -- BuzzFeed website - Buzzfeed News   12/8/2015

112   (book) Wildness and sensation: An anthropology of sinister and sensuous realms -- Chapter: the social life of faeces - System in the Dirt
Sjaak van der Geest
Emeritus Professor of Medical Anthropology at the University of Amsterdam

113   (book) Michael O'Mara Books, 1997
Thunder, Flush and Thomas Crapper
Adam Hart-Davis

114   https://soranews24.com/2012/11/23/a-frank-discussion-about-anuses-and-why-washlet-toilets-may-be-bad-for-your-health/
A Frank Discussion About Anuses and Why Washlet Toilets May be Bad For Your Health -- Philip Kendall   Nov 23, 2012
Sora News 24 - Bringing you yesterday's news from Japan and Asia, today.

115   World J Urol. 1999 Jun;17(3):145-50
Some historical aspects of urinals and urine receptacles.
Mattelaer JJ.
Department of Urology, CAZK Groeninghe, Kortrijk, Belgium.

116   Gesundheitswesen. 1992 Aug;54(8):410-6
[Construction hygiene in the area of bathing and recreation][Article in German]
Sonntag HG.
Abteilung Hygiene und Medizinische Mikrobiologie-Hygiene-Institut, Universitat
Heidelberg.

117   http://www.earthisland.org/journal/index.php/magazine/entry/
not_a_square_to_spare
Not a Square to Spare, Toilet paper, it turns out, grows on trees
NOELLE ROBBINS AUTUMN 2010 -- Earth Island Journal website

118   Soc Hist Med. 2000 Apr;13(1):63-85
Profit is a dirty word - the development of the public baths and wash-houses in
Britain 1847-1915. -- Sheard S.
Dept of Public Health and School of History, University of Liverpool, UK.

119   The Dollar Shave Club website
The Very Absorbing History of Toilet Paper
C. BRIAN SMITH

120   J Water Health. 2018 Jun;16(3):346-358. doi: 10.2166/wh.2017.137.
Microorganism levels in spray from warm-water bidet toilet seats - factors
affecting total viable and heterotrophic plate counts, and examination of the
fluctuations and origins of Pseudomonas aeruginosa.
Iyo T1, Asakura K2, Nakano M3, Omae K3.
Department of Health Sciences, School of Allied Health Sciences, Kitasato
University, Japan

121   (Book) W. W. Norton & Co Inc 1950
Psychosomatic Medicine, page 117
Franz Alexander MD

122 http://www.portapotty.net/plumbing/
The History of Modern Plumbing: 20 important indoor plumbing milestones
Porta-Potty website

123   Metropolitan Books, Henry Holt and Company, Jul 7, 2009
The Big Necessity: The Unmentionable World of Human Waste and Why It
Matters
Rose George

124   Material from the former Toto website that was too good to leave out. Toto
is so successful that they no longer need to include testimonials in their current
website. Besides they get a ton of testimonials free from their listings on Amazon,
some of which are included in this book. This material is no longer on the web,
but was well cited in the original, published in 2004.

125   IOS Press, 2011
 A Friendly Rest Room: Developing Toilets of the Future for Disabled and Elderly
People -- [book chapter] Alla Turca: Squatting for Health and Hygiene
Oya DEMIRBILEK -- J.F.M. Molenbroek et al. (Eds.)
University of New South Wales, Sydney, Australia

126   Nursing & Residential Care, August 2005, Vol 7, No 8
Providing convenient and accessible toilet facilities
Julie Swann -- Julie Swann is an independent occupational therapist

127   https://my.clevelandclinic.org/health/articles/4089-dermatitis
Cleveland Clinic Web article: Dermatitis

128   https://clean4happy.com/8-things-to-keep-your-septic-system-from-failing/
8 Things To Keep Your Septic System From Failing
Dan Harris January 23, 2018 -- Clean 4 Happy product reviews website

129   Clinics in Colon and Rectal Surgery 2016; 29(01): 038-042
Pruritus Ani -- Parswa Ansari
Hofstra North Shore-LIJ School of Medicine, Lenox Hill Hospital, New York

130   Elsevier Health Sciences, Nov 7, 2013 - 544 pages
Older People: Issues and Innovations in Care
Rhonda Nay, Sally Garratt, Deirdre Fetherstonhaugh

131   J Korean Med Sci. 2011 Jan; 26(1): 71–77.
Effect of Electronic Toilet System (Bidet) on Anorectal Pressure in Normal Healthy Volunteers - Influence of Different Types of Water Stream and Temperature
Seungbum Ryoo,1 Yoon Suk Song,1 Mi Sun Seo,1 Heung-Kwon Oh,1 etal
Department of Surgery, Seoul National University College of Medicine, Seoul, Korea

132   https://www.verywellhealth.com/how-to-take-a-sitz-bath-1944927
Web article: How to Take a Sitz Bath
Barbara Bolen, PhD
Very Well Health website

133   Techniques in Coloproctology, September 2015, Volume 19, Issue 9, pp 535–540
Comparison between a new electronic bidet and conventional sitz baths: a manometric evaluation of the anal resting pressure in normal healthy volunteers
S.-B. RyooH.-K. OhE. C. HanY. S. SongM. S. SeoE. K. Choe etal
Division of Colorectal Surgery, Department of Surgery, Seoul National University

134 National Research Institute for Child Health and Development, Tokyo Japan
A Japanese study on childhood leukemia in relation to the use of electric appliances
Tomohiro Saito 1, Michinori Kabuto2, Hiroshi Nitta2, etal
National Research Institute for Child Health and Development, Tokyo, Japan

135   Ostomy Wound Manage. 1996 Aug;42(7):28-30, 32-4, 36-7.
Perineal skin injury: extrinsic environmental risk factors.
Faria DT, Shwayder T, Krull EA.

136   Clinical Journal of Oncology Nursing . Jan/Feb2000, Vol. 4 Issue 1, p15-21. 7p.
A Nursing Protocol for the Management of Perineal-Rectal Skin Alterations.
Haisfield-Wolfe, Mary Ellen; Rund, Cecilia

137   BJS Volume 86, Issue10, 1 October 1999, Pages 1337-1340
Treatment of persistent pruritus ani in a combined colorectal and dermatological clinic

S. Dasan S. M. Neill D. R. Donaldson Mr H. J. Scott
Dept of Colorectal Surgery and Dermatology, St Peter's Hospital, Surrey UK

138   Diseases of the Colon & Rectum May 1982, Volume 25, Issue 4, pp 358–363
Prospective studies on the etiology and treatment of pruritus ani
Lee E. SmithDean HenrichsRobert D. McCullah
Division of Colon and Rectal Surgery Uniformed Services University of the
Health Sciences, National Naval Medical Center, Bethesda MD

139   Postgraduate Medicine Pages 76-80 Published online: 16 May 2016
Pruritus ani - Practical therapy for persistent itching
Edsel J. Aucoin , MD

140   Postgraduate Medicine Volume 77, 1985 - Issue 1
Pruritus ani - What to do, what not to do to control this infernal itch
John Alexander-Williams , MD, FRCS, FACS

141   https://en.wikipedia.org/wiki/Anal_fissure#Causes
Web article, "Anal fissure"
Wikipedia public encyclopedia

142   Dermatology. 1997;195(3):258-62
 Effects of soap and detergents on skin surface pH, stratum corneum hydration
and fat content in infants
Gfatter R, Hackl P, Braun F.
Department of Pediatrics, University of Vienna, School of Medicine, Austria

143   Ostomy Wound Manage. 1996 Apr;42(3):32-4, 36, 38-40, passim.
Breaking the cycle: the etiology of incontinence dermatitis and evaluating and
using skin care products.
Fiers SA.

144   World J Gastroenterol. 2004 Mar 1; 10(5): 713–716.
An extended assessment of bowel habits in a general population
Gabrio Bassotti, Massimo Bellini, Filippo Pucciani, etal
Sezione di Gastroenterologia ed Epatologia, Dipartimento di Medicina Clinica e
Sperimentale, Università di Perugia

145   Z Gastroenterol. 1992 Jan;30(1):24-34.
[Behavior therapy in gastrointestinal functional disorders] [Article in German]
Cuntz U1, Pollmann H, Enck P. Klinik Niederrhein, Bad Neuenahr.

146   Digestive Diseases and Sciences September 1993, Volume 38, Issue 9, pp 1569–1580
U. S. Householder survey of functional gastrointestinal disorders - Prevalence,
sociodemography, and health impact
Douglas A. Drossman, Zhiming Li, Eileen Andruzzi, et al

147   Digestive Diseases and Sciences August 1987, Volume 32, Issue 8, pp 841–845
Bowel habits in young adults not seeking health care
Robert S. Sandler, Douglas A. Drossman
Division of Digestive Diseases and Nutrition, and the Core Center in Diarrheal
Diseases, University of North Carolina School of Medicine, Chapel Hill

148   American Journal of Physical Medicine & Rehabilitation: March 2007 -
Volume 86 - Issue 3 - pp 200-204

A Washing Toilet Seat with a CCD Camera Monitor to Stimulate Bowel Movement in Patients with Spinal Cord Injury
Uchikawa, Ken MD; Takahashi, Hidetoshi MD, PhD; Deguchi, etal
Department of Rehabilitation Medicine, National Hospital Organization, Murayama Medical Center, Tokyo, Japan

149   Neth J Surg. 1991;43(6):213-7.
Functional constipation - results of application of the colorectal laboratory.
Kuijpers JH1.
Department of Surgery, Academic Hospital St. Radboud, Catholic University, Nijmegen, The Netherlands.

150   NATURE REVIEWS | DISEASE PRIMERS VOLUME 3 | ARTICLE
 NUMBER 17095
Chronic constipation
Michael Camilleri1, Alexander C. Ford2, Gary M. Mawe3, et al
Division of Gastroenterology and Hepatology, Mayo Clinic College of Medicine and Science, Rochester, MN USA

151   https://www.aqualibria.com/colonic-irrigation-resources/colon-hydrotherapy-constipation/
Colon Hydrotherapy and its clinical applications (part 3)
Donald J. Mantell, M.D.
Professional Member AANC   Duplicate of 277

152   J Neurogastroenterol Motil, Vol. 22 No. 4 October, 2016
Prevalence and Self-recognition of Chronic Constipation - Results of an Internet Survey
Akio Tamura, Toshihiko Tomita, Tadayuki Oshima, Fumihiko Toyoshima, et al
Division of Gastroenterology, Department of Internal Medicine, Hyogo College of Medicine, Hyogo, Japan

153   J Am Geriatr Soc. 1989 May;37(5):423-9.
Constipation in the elderly living at home. Definition, prevalence, and relationship to lifestyle and health status.
Whitehead WE, Drinkwater D, Cheskin LJ, Heller BR, Schuster MM.
Johns Hopkins University School of Medicine, Baltimore, Maryland

154   J Korean Acad Fundam Nurs Vol.20 No.4, 333-344, November, 2013
Prevalence and Factors Influencing Constipation in School Age Children
Ji Hyun Park, Jung Tae Son
Medical Science Nursing, Nursing Science, Geriatrics, Catholic University of Daegu

155   Gastroenterology Clinics of North America Volume 30, Issue 1, 1 March 2001, Pages 97-114
DYSSYNERGIC DEFECATION
Satish S.C., RaoMD, PhD, FRCP(LON)
Section of Neurogastroenterology, Division of Gastroenterology-Hepatology, Department of Internal Medicine, University of Iowa College of Medicine, Iowa City, Iowa

156   J Korean Med Sci. 2011 Jan; 26(1): 71–77.
Effect of Electronic Toilet System (Bidet) on Anorectal Pressure in Normal Healthy Volunteers: Influence of Different Types of Water Stream and Temperature
Seungbum Ryoo,1 Yoon Suk Song,1 Mi Sun Seo,1 Heung-Kwon Oh, et al
1Department of Surgery, Seoul National University College of Medicine, Seoul, Korea.

157   https://en.wikipedia.org/wiki/Diarrhea
Web article, "Diarrhea"
Wikipedia online public encyclopedia

158   The American Journal of Gastroenterology Volume 98, Issue 4, April 2003, Pages 789-797
Does psychological distress modulate functional gastrointestinal symptoms and health care seeking? A prospective, community cohort study
Natasha AKoloski, Nicholas JTalleyM.D, MBoyceM.D.
Department of Medicine, University of Sydney, Nepean Hospital, Penrith NSW, Australia

159   Am J Gastroenterol. 2004 Feb;99(2):350-7.
Psychosocial factors are linked to functional gastrointestinal disorders - a population based nested case-control study.
Locke GR, Weaver AL, Melton LJ, Talley NJ.
Division of Gastroenterology and Internal Medicine, Department of Health Sciences Research, Mayo Clinic, Rochester, MN

160   Psychiatric Services 49:951–955, 1998
Functional Impairment Associated With Psychological Distress and Medical Severity in Rural Primary Care Patients
Alisabeth Thurston-Hicks, M.D. Susan Paine, M.P.H. Michael Hollifield, M.D

161   Dig Dis Sci. 1996 Apr;41(4):633-40.
Gastrointestinal symptoms and psychiatric disorders in the general population. Findings from NIMH Epidemiologic Catchment Area Project.
North CS, Alpers DH, Thompson SJ, Spitznagel EL.
Depts of Psychiatry and Internal Medicine Washington University School of Medicine, St. Louis

162   Gut, 1988, 29, 17-20
Urological abnormalities in young women with severe constipation
J J BANNISTER, W T LAWRENCE, A SMITH, D G THOMAS, etal
Department of Surgery and Sub-Dept of Human Gastrointestinal Physiology and Nutrition, Royal Hallamshire Hospital, Sheffield,

163   Int J Colorectal Dis. 1988 Nov;3(4):207-9.
Function of the striated anal sphincter during straining in control subjects and constipated patients with a radiologically normal rectum or idiopathic megacolon.
Barnes PR1, Lennard-Jones JE. -- St. Mark's Hospital, London, UK.

164   The Jennings Hygeia bidet website – www.southernbidet.com

Wayne Jennings and his Hygeia bidet are now retired. Website is now gone, but this remains a good personal message on how Wayne used his bidet:

165   GASTROENTEROLOGY 1986;90:53
Impairment of Defecation in Young Women With Severe Constipation
N. W. READ, J. M. TIMMS, L. J. BARFIELD, etal
Department of Surgery, Royal Hallamshire Hospital, Sheffield, UK

166   Baillieres Clin Gastroenterol. 1992 Mar;6(1):179-91.
Testing for and the role of anal and rectal sensation.
Rogers J.

167   Ital J Gastroenterol. 1991 Nov;23(8 Suppl 1):10-2.
Constipation: physiopathology and classification
Miglioli M1.
Cattedra di Terapia Medica Sistematica, Policlinico S. Orsola, Bologna, Italy.

168   Int J Colorectal Dis. 1986 Jul;1(3):175-82.
Physiological studies in young women with chronic constipation.
Bannister JJ, Timms JM, Barfield LJ, Donnelly TC, Read NW.
Clinical Research Unit, H FloorRoyal Hallamshire Hospital, Sheffield UK

169   Gut, 1990, 31, 1056-1061
Relation between rectal sensation and anal function in normal subjects and patients with faecal incontinence
W M Sun, N W Read, P B Miner
Subdepartment of Human Gastrointestinal Physiology and Nutrition, Royal Hallamshire Hospital, University of Sheffield

170   J Korean Med Sci. 2011 Jan; 26(1): 71–77.
Effect of Electronic Toilet System (Bidet) on Anorectal Pressure in Normal Healthy Volunteers - Influence of Different Types of Water Stream and Temperature
Seungbum Ryoo,1 Yoon Suk Song,1 Mi Sun Seo,1 Heung-Kwon Oh, etal
Department of Surgery, Seoul National University College of Medicine, Korea.

171 https://childrensmd.org/browse-by-age-group/toddler-pre-school/diarrhea-diaster-managing-menace/
Children's MD website, "Diarrhea Disaster: Managing a Menace"
Kirstin Campbell, M.D
Instructor of Pediatrics at Washington University School of Medicine

172   https://en.wikipedia.org/wiki/Lactose_intolerance
Web article, "Lactose Intolerance"
Wikipedia public online encyclopedia

173 https://www.mayoclinic.org/diseases-conditions/fecal-incontinence/symptoms -causes/syc-20351397
Mayo Clinic website, "Fecal Incontinence" April 17 2019
Mayo Clinic staff

174 https://www.proremodeler.com/bidets-finally-making-inroads-us-bathrooms
Bidets Finally Making Inroads in US Bathrooms:
Pro Remodeler Magazine January 27, 2017

175   J Gerontol Nurs. 1989 May;15(5):16-23
Incontinence
Heller BR, Whitehead WE, Johnson LD.

176   Med J Aust. 2002 Jan 21;176(2):54-7
Prevalence of faecal incontinence and associated risk factors; an underdiagnosed problem in the Australian community?
Kalantar JS, Howell S, Talley NJ.
Department of Medicine, The University of Sydney, Nepean Hospital, Australia

177   Journal of Pediatric Surgery, Vol31, No 4 (April), 1996: pp 563.667
Coping Strategies of Children With Faecal Incontinence
Lorraine Ludman, Lewis Spitz
Department of Paediatric Surgery, Institute of Child Health and Great Ormond Street Hospital for Children, London, England.

178   A thesis submitted to fulfil requirements for the degree of Doctor of Philosophy 2018
The clinical utility of the electronic toilet-top bidet for Australian nursing home residents and staff
Meredith Gresham
Ageing Work and Health Research Unit, Faculty of Health Sciences, University of Sydney

179   https://www.cigna.com/individuals-families/health-wellness/hw/medical-topics/hydrotherapy -tr3554spec
Website article: "What is hydrotherapy?" November 29, 2017
Author: Healthwise Staff   Medical Review: Adam Husney, MD
CIGNA INTERNATIONAL HEALTH INSURANCE

180   https://www.aqualibria.com/colonic-irrigation-resources/colon-hydrotherapy- conditions/
Colon Hydrotherapy and its clinical applications (part 6)
Donald J. Mantell, M.D. (Professional Member AANC)
Aqualiberia website - Colon Hydrotherapy Media spa

181   Dis Colon Rectum. 1997 Jul;40(7):802-5.
Clinical value of colonic irrigation in patients with continence disturbances.
Briel JW1, Schouten WR, Vlot EA, Smits S, van Kessel I.
Department of General Surgery, University Hospital Dijkzigt, Rotterdam, The Netherlands.

182   Diseases of the Colon & Rectum: July-August 1959 - Volume 2 - Issue 4 - ppg 335-336
Guest Editorial, In Praise of the Bidet
Pack George T. M.D.
Pack was a doctor widely recognized for his achievements in oncology

183   http://www.portable-bidet.com/benefits.asp?page=4
Bidet Benefits
Personal+Hygeine Systems website sells bidets

184   http://factsanddetails.com/japan/cat19/sub121/item643.html#chapter-2
Facts and Details Blog, "Toilets in Japan" 2009

History of Toilets in Japan, High Tech Toilets in Japan
Jeffrey Hays -- Facts and Details Website

185   Gastroenterol Hepatol (N Y). 2014 May; 10(5): 294–301.
Common Anorectal Disorders
Amy E. Foxx-Orenstein, DO, Sarah B. Umar, MD, Michael D. Crowell, PhD
Division of Gastroenterology at the Mayo Clinic in Scottsdale, Arizona.

186   http://www.hemorrhoid.net/hemorrhoids.php
What Are Hemorrhoids?
Hemorrhoid & Rectal Disease Information & Treatment Centers.

187   https://www.bidet.org/pages/bidets-for-health-issues
Bidets For 9 Common Health Issues, "Hemmorhoids"
Bidet.org is an online seller of bidets

188   https://www.bidet.org/blogs/news/how-to-clean-a-bidet
Bidet.org website, "How To Clean A Bidet" Aug 16, 2018
Bidet.org is an online seller of bidets

189   Preventive Medicine Reports Volume 6, June 2017, Pages 121-Bidet toilet
use and incidence of hemorrhoids or urogenital infections - A one-year follow-up
web survey
TeppeiKiuchiaKeikoAsakurabMakikoNakanoaKazuyukiOmaea
Department of Preventive Medicine and Public Health, School of Medicine, Keio
University, Japan

190   https://www.reddit.com/r/funny/comments/1m0boz/
Reddit website - r/funny

191   https://www.aad.org/public/skin-hair-nails/anti-aging-skin-care/causes-
of-aging-skin
American Academy of Dermatology website
"Anti-aging skin care" 11 ways to reduce premature skin aging

192   J Gerontol Nurs. 1996 May;22(5):10-8
What can you do about your patient's dry skin?
Hardy MA.

193   https://www.sanitary-net.com/global/asking_specialists/interview01.html
Toilet Navigation - Women Ask the Specialists How to use a spray seat properly
Dr. Maki Nakata
consultant obsterician-gynecologist at Mitsui Memorial Hospital

194   https://medlineplus.gov/ency/article/000862.htm
Medline Plus Encyclopedia, "Balanitis"

195 https://www.mayoclinic.org/diseases-conditions/kidney-infection/
symptoms-causes/syc-20353387
Mayo Clinic website: Kidney Infection

196   https://www.mayoclinic.org/search/search-results?q=cystitis
Mayo Clinic website, "Interstitial Cystitis"

197   https://medlineplus.gov/ency/article/000439.htm
Medline Plus Encyclopedia, "Urethritis"

198   https://medlineplus.gov/vaginitis.html
US NIH, Medline Plus encyclopedia, "Vaginitis"

199   The Journal of Obstetrics and Gynaecology ResearchVolume 36, Issue 5, October 2010, Pages 1071–1074
Habitual use of warm-water cleaning toilets is related to the aggravation of vaginal microflora
Mitsuharu Ogino, Koichi Iino, Shigeki Minoura

200   Reviews in Medical Microbiology: July 2016 - Volume 27 - Issue 3 - p 87–94
Probiotics for treating bacterial vaginosis
Mogha, Kanchan V. Prajapati, Jashbhai B.

201   Journal of Obstetric, Gynecologic, & Neonatal Nursing May 2003 Volume 32, Issue 3, Pages 287–296
Prevention and Treatment of Vulvovaginal Candidiasis Using Exogenous Lactobacillus
Heather S. Jeavons, MSN, APRN- C, RNC

202 https://www.verywellhealth.com/avoid-skin-trauma-to-minimize-psoriasis-2788293
Avoid Skin Trauma to Minimize Psoriasis
Dean Goodless, MD
Verywell website: Updated August 08, 2018

203   Internal Medicine Vol. 42, No. 4 (April 2003)
Urinary Bladder Infection/Irritation among Female Users of a High-Tech Toilet
Isao MiYOSHl, Taeko MiTSUOKAand Hirokuni Taguchi
Third Department of Medicine, Kochi Medical School, Kochi

204   Preventive Medicine Reports Volume 6, June 2017, Pages 121-125
Bidet toilet use and incidence of hemorrhoids or urogenital infections - A one-year follow-up web survey
TeppeiKiuchiaKeikoAsakurabMakikoNakanoaKazuyukiOmaea
Department of Preventive Medicine and Public Health, School of Medicine, Keio University, Tokyo, Japan

205   Epidemiology & Infection Volume 146, Issue 6 April 2018 , pp. 763-770
Relationship between bidet toilet use and haemorrhoids and urogenital infections - a 3-year follow-up web survey
K. Asakura (a1) (a2), M. Nakano (a2) and K. Omae (a2)
Department of Environmental and Occupational Health, School of Medicine, Toho University, Tokyo, Japan

206   Hinyokika Kiyo. Acta Urologica Japonica [2016, 62(2):53-56]
[The User Fact-Finding on the Electric Warm-Water Lavage Toilet Seats in the Women Consulting Our Urological Outpatient Clinic].
Hongoh S , Usui Y , Inatuchi H , Fujisaki A , Kinjo M etal
The Department of Urology, Yotsuya Medical Cube.

207   Mayo Clin Proc. 1982 Mar;57(3):185-8.
Primary closure and continuous irrigation of the perineal wound after proctectomy
Waits JO, Dozois RR, Kelly KA.

208   https://www.angieslist.com/articles/americans-slowly-embrace-bidet.htm
Angie's List Website: Americans slowly embrace the bidet
Matthew Brady - Date Published: Jul 16 2009

209   Compend Contin Ed Dent 2018; 39(Suppl. 2):8-13.
Waterpik® Water Flosser: Safe and Effective up to 100 psi
Goyal CR, Lyle DM, Qaqish JG, Schuller R.

210   Ostomy Wound Manage. 2000 Apr;46(4):44-9.
Pulsed lavage: promoting comfort and healing in home care.
Morgan D1, Hoelscher J.
Lifespan Home and Hospice Care, Battle Creek, Michigan

211   Ostomy Wound Manage. 2007 Apr;53(4):64-6, 68-70, 72.
Comparison of wound irrigation and tangential hydrodissection in bacterial clearance of contaminated wounds: results of a randomized, controlled clinical study. -- Granick MS1, Tenenhaus M, Knox KR, Ulm JP.
Division of Plastic Surgery, University of Medicine and Dentistry of New Jersey, New Jersey Medical School, Newark

212   NRDC www.laondaverde.org/media/pressreleases/041118b.asp
KIMBERLY-CLARK: CUTTING DOWN ANCIENT FORESTS TO MAKE THROWAWAY PRODUCTS
Susan Casey-Lefkowitz
Natural Resources Defense Council

213   Dis Colon Rectum. 2005 Dec;48(12):2336-40.
Sitz bath: where is the evidence? Scientific basis of a common practice.
Tejirian T1, Abbas MA.
Department of Surgery, Section of Colon and Rectal Surgery, Kaiser Permanente, Los Angeles, CA

214   ANZ Journal of Surgery Volume78, Issue5 May 2008 Pages 398-401
WARM SITZ BATH DOES NOT REDUCE SYMPTOMS IN POSTHAEMORRHOIDECTOMY PERIOD: A RANDOMIZED, CONTROLLED STUDY
Pravin J. Gupta

215   www.theinfolist.com/php/SummaryGet.php?FindGo=Paper%20industry
The InfoList website: The Paper Industry
Stephen Payne

216   https://vagabondish.com/an-idiots-incomplete-guide-to-the-bidet/
An Idiot's Incomplete Guide to the Bidet
Christopher Cook
Vagabondish website: Adventurous travel for semi-responsible adults

217   https://www.mamavation.com/brands/toilet-paper.html
How Toxic Is Your Toilet Paper? Investigation of Brands
Mamavation website

218   Int J Clin Pharmacol Ther. 2003 Jan;41(1):14-21
 Differential therapy of constipation--a review.
Wanitschke R, Goerg KJ, Loew D.I.

Medizinische Klinik und Poliklinik, Johannes Gutenberg-Universitat, Mainz, Germany.

219   ITALIAN JOURNAL OF GYNAECOLOGY & OBSTETRICS 1994
The perineal flora of women according to their method of genital cleansing
SEMPRINI, AUGUSTO ENRICO (Primo), SAVASI, VALERIA MARIA
University of Milan | UNIMI · Department of Biomedical and Clinical Sciences

220   https://www.hayksaakian.com/when-was-toilet-paper-invented/
When Was Toilet Paper Invented? We Explain The History
hayk | Nov 14, 2018
Who Invented Toilet Paper?

221   https://www.nachi.org/bidets.htm
International Association of Certified Home Inspectors

222   https://www.risiinfo.com/product/exploding-chinese-tissue-business-opportunities-challenges/
Exploding Chinese Tissue Business – Opportunities and Challenges
FastMarkets RISI website

223   https://www.papnews.com/insight/global-tissue-outlook-strong-demand-growth-led-emerging- markets/
Strong demand growth led by Emerging Markets
Global Tissue Outlook

224   https://www.statista.com/outlook/80010000/109/toilet-paper/united-states
Toilet Paper revenue
Statista website: The Portal for Statistics

225   https://www.nrdc.org/sites/default/files/issue-tissue-how-americans-are-flushing-forests-down-toilet-report.pdf
The Issue With Tissue - How Americans are flushing forest down the toilet (2019)
Jennifer Skene, with significant contributions from Shelley Vinyard
Natural Resources Defense Council (NRDC) website

226   https://www.reddit.com/r/funny/comments/1m0boz/
Reddit website - r/funny
i_bought_a_bidet_3_months_ago_and_havent_pooped/

227   http://in.rediff.com/news/2001/jul/07maneka.htm
Exchanging Life for Toilet Paper? -- Maneka Gandhi
(India) Union minister of state for social justice and empowerment.
Rediff website - Guest Column - July 7, 2001

228   https://www.yahoo.com/beauty/bidets-are-healthier-than-toilet-paper-so-why-111571549767.html
Bidets Are Healthier Than Toilet Paper. So Why Don't We Use Them?
Yahoo Beauty: Health•February 24, 2015 -

229   https://dl.acm.org/citation.cfm?id=3038420
ACM Digital Library: Initial Interaction Concept for a Robotic Toilet System
Paul Panek, Peter Mayer

230   https://www.smh.com.au/lifestyle/flushing-our-future-down-the-toilet-20131104-2wvg1.html
Flushing our future down the toilet
Sam de Brito
The Sydney Morning Herald Newspaper 4 November 2013

231   https://www.betterplanetpaper.com/uearn2/Paper-Awareness
Roll Out The Paper Stats!
Better Planet website

232   https://www.statista.com/outlook/80010000/109/toilet-paper/united-states
Toilet Paper revenue
Statista – the Statistics Portal website

233   Bioresource Technology Volume 77, Issue 3, May 2001, Pages 275-286
The treatment of pulp and paper mill effluent: a review
GThompson, JSwain, MKay, C.FForstera

234   Forum for Social Economics, DOI: 10.1080/07360932.2017.1387864
From Primitive Accumulation to Modernized Poverty - Examining Flush toilets through the Four Invaluation Processes
Alexander Dunlap
Department of Social and Cultural Anthropology, Vrije Universiteit Amsterdam, Amsterdam, Netherlands

235   https://www.amazon.com/Woodbridge-Elongated-Temperature-Controlled-Functions/dp/B07XCMV19F/ref=sr_1_1?keywords=WOODBRIDGE+Luxury+Elongated+T-0737&qid=1572858526&sr=8-1
Amazon Questions about WOODBRIDGE Luxury Elongated One Piece Advanced Smart Seat with Temperature Controlled Wash Functions and Air Dryer, Toilet with Bidet. T-0737

236   https://www.mayoclinic.org/diseases-conditions/hemorrhoids/symptoms-causes/syc-20360268
Hemorrhoids
Advice from the Facts and Details Blog, Mayo Clinic website

237   Int J Clin Pract, November 2014, 68, 11, 1388–1399.
Therapeutic management of anal eczema - an evidence-based review
B. Havlickova, G. H. Weyandt

238   International Journal of Surgery and Surgical Sciences Vol 3, No 3 (2015)
SITZ BATH IN POST OPERATIVE CASES OF HAEMORRHOIDS - IS IT USEFUL ? -- Vishal Dubey, Ritesh Dixit

239   http://www.worldwatch.org/node/5142
Matters of Scale - Into the Toilet
Worldwatch Institute website

240   https://www.risiinfo.com/product/exploding-chinese-tissue-business-opportunities-challenges/
Exploding Chinese Tissue Business – Opportunities and Challenges
FastMarkets RISI website

241   https://www.southeastgreen.com/index.php/seg-features/tips-a-faqs/tips-to-green-your-life/10551-how-much-toilet-paper-is-used-per-year
How Much Toilet Paper Is Used Per Year?
SAM THOMPSON   -- SouthEast Green website 01 FEBRUARY 2014

242   https://www.betterplanetpaper.com/CorpOrphan/Paper-Awareness
EVERYONE WIPES! WE ALL WIPE SOMETHING, SOMEWHERE.
Better Planet Paper Company website: "Roll out the Paper Stats"

243   https://europeantissue.com/pdfs/060630-TGTF,%203moist%20tissue%20development,%20update%20060719.pdf
The Moist Toilet Tissue Opportunity
European Tissue Symposium

244   https://europeantissue.com/pdfs/060630-TGTF,%202france%20premium%20segment_%20moltonel_%20gp.pdf
How Moltonel Succeeded in Creating a Premium Quality New Segment in the French Toilet Paper Market: Moltonel's "Thick, Strong and Soft" Toilet Paper Has Created a New Premium Quality Segment in The French Toilet Paper Market
European Tissue Symposium

245   https://www.papnews.com/insight/global-tissue-outlook-strong-demand-growth-led-emerging-markets/
Global Tissue Outlook Strong demand growth led by Emerging Markets
PapNews – News From the Paper Industry Sector

246   https://www.reddit.com/r/BuyItForLife/comments/3mj73v/can_someone_recommend_a_bidet/
Can someone recommend a bidet?
Reddit website

247   https://rinseworks.com/reviews-2
Aquaus handheld bidet website - Reviews

248   https://superiorbidet.com/testimonials/
Superior Bidet Website - Testimonials

249   https://www.washingtonpost.com/news/wonk/wp/2015/03/13/what-the-rise-of-luxury-toilet-paper-says-about-the-economy/?noredirect=on&utm_term=.15b72e94858c
Economic Policy: The rise of luxury toilet paper
Drew Harwell   -- The Washington Post website March 13, 2015

250 https://www.tissuestory.com/2018/04/26/market-pulp-tissue-has-become-the-biggest-global-buyer/
Market pulp: Tissue has become the biggest global buyer
HUGH BUSINESS
Tissue Story website: The Global Knowledge Center for Tissue Paper Products

251 https://www.tissuestory.com/2019/01/21/tissuestory-profile-patrick-boateng-issue-category-buyer-kroger-company/
TissueStory profile: Patrick Boateng, Tissue category buyer, Kroger Company
The Tissue Story website

252 https://www.museumoflondon.org.uk/discover/exhibiting-fatberg
monster-whitechapel
Fatberg! Exhibiting the 'Monster of Whitechapel'
Museum of London website

253 https://en.wikipedia.org/wiki/Wet_wipe#Effect_on_sewage_systems
Wet Wipe
Wikipedia online encyclopedia

254 https://www.hgtv.com/design/rooms/bathrooms/euro-style-
personal-hygiene-with-the-bidet
The bidet: What is this mysterious French lavatory fixture, and will it ever find a
place in American bathrooms? -- John Yates
HGTV website, Euro-style Personal Hygiene With the Bidet (2019)

255 http://upstartpower.com/2018/05/how-much-electricity-does-an-average-
home-need/
How much electricity does an average home need?
BY ROBERTBOOKER -- Upstart Power blog: MAY 29, 2018

256 Ergonomics in Design: The Quarterly of Human Factors Applications April
2015 vol. 23 no. 2 16-22
Work Postures When Assisting People at the Toilet
Jenny Hjalmarson, Stefan Lundberg

257 http://newoldage.blogs.nytimes.com/2012/03/27/begin-the-bidet/?_r=0
New York Times website -- Begin the Bidet
PAULA SPAN MARCH 27, 2012

258   https://www.tissuestory.com/2017/03/12/tissue-a-social-environmental-
and-economic-sustainability-star/
Tissue: A Social, Environmental and Economic Sustainability Star
Suhas Apte and Tim McFarland -- Tissue Story website blog

259 https://www.theatlantic.com/technology/archive/2015/09/americas-
sewage-crisis-public-health/405541/
TECHNOLOGY, "Flushing the Toilet Has Never Been Riskier"
MARY ANNA EVANS
The Atlantic Magazine website SEP 17, 2015

260 https://www.jerseywaterworks.org/wp-content/uploads/2018/08/NJ-
CSOs-Fact-Sheet-UPDATED.pdf
New Jersey Combined Sewer System Fact Sheet

261 https://www.homeadvisor.com/cost/plumbing/install-a-septic-tank/
How Much Does A Septic System Cost?
Home Advisor website

262 Sewage Tratement Plant Construction cost Index 1963
Construction Categories, Components, Costs and Percent of costs for a 1.0 High
Rate Trickling Filter Plant Kansas City MO-August 1962
Total Plant cost $462,000
US Dept HEW, Public health Service Publication 1069

263   https://www.samcotech.com/cost-wastewater-treatment-system/
How Much Does a Wastewater Treatment System Cost? (Pricing, Factores, Etc.)
Samco website 2016

264   https://www.commercialappeal.com/story/news/2018/12/10/shelby-county-sewer-system-unincorporated-areas/2231570002/
Shelby County scraps sewer plan with $35 million price tag
Katherine Burgess
Memphis Commercial Appeal website Dec. 10, 2018

265   https://www.buzzfeed.com/terripous/what-is-the-family-cloth-and-why-should-you-use-it-an
What Is "The Family Cloth"? And "Why Do People Use It?" An Explainer
Terri Pous -- Buzzfeed website March 8, 2018

266   https://www.greenpeace.org/usa/destroying-forests-to-make-toilet-paper-is-worse-than-driving-hummers/
Destroying forests to make toilet paper is "worse than driving Hummers"
Lindsey Allen -- Greenpeace website February 26, 2009

267   Ergonomics in Design: The Quarterly of Human Factors Applications
April 2015 vol. 23 no. 2 16-22
Work Postures When Assisting People at the Toilet
Jenny Hjalmarson, Stefan Lundberg

268   Ramdom House Books, Volume 1, Part 3, Page 33
Studies in the Psychology of Sex 1936
(mentioned in Kura's book The Bathroom)

269   (book) SpringerBriefs in Environmental Science. 2014
Biological Odour Treatment.
(chapter) Emissions from Pulping
Bajpai P.

270   (book) Chelsea Green publishing
Holy Shit: Managing Manure to Save Mankind
Gene Logsdon
He has researched and written over two dozen books on traditional agriculture, and practices what he preaches. Former staff at Organic Gardening magazine

271   https://en.m.wikipedia.org/wiki/Environmental_impact_of_paper
Environmental Impact of Paper
Wikipedia online encyclopedia

272   https://www.newsmax.com/health/health-news/infections-hand-fist-bump/2014/01/09/id/546258/
CDC: 80 Percent of Infections Spread by Hands
Newsmax website   09 January 2014

273   electronic journal of contemporary japanese studies   Volume 16, Issue 3 (Article 8 in 2016).
From\ Night Soil to Washlet-The Material Culture of Japanese Toilets
Marta E. Szczygiel -- Graduate School of Human Sciences, Osaka University

274 http://www.bohotravel.org/2016/08/28/bidet/
The Boho Traveler blog: Free spirit, Nomadic Toes: What is a Bidet?
Sydney Zaruba August 28, 2016

275 https://en.wikipedia.org/wiki/Durable_medical_equipment Division=1710
Wikipedia online encyclopedia article, "Durable Medical Equipment"

276 https://www.mayoclinic.org/diseases-conditions/urinary-tract-infection/
symptoms-causes/syc-20353447
Mayo Clinic website -- Urinary tract infection (UTI)

277 http://www.colonhealth.net/colon_hydrotherapy/mantell6.htm
Colon Hydrotherapy and its Clinical Applications: Colon hydrotherapy prevents
build up of bacterial toxins in the lymphatic system and colon
Donald J. Mantell, M.D. -- Professional Member AANC
The Colon Therapist's Network Website December 10, 2018

278 https://theconversation.com/why-children-find-poo-so-hilarious-and-how-
adults-should-tackle-it-72258
Why children find 'poo' so hilarious - and how adults should tackle it
Justin H G Williams
Senior Clinical Lecturer in Child Psychiatry, University of Aberdeen
The Conversation website February 2, 2017

279 https://www.health.harvard.edu/staying-healthy/managing_common_
vulvar_skin_conditions
Managing common vulvar skin conditions
Harvard Health Publishing website

280 https://uihc.org/health-topics/vulvar-skin-care-guidelines
Vulvar skin care guidelines
University of Iowa Hospitals and Clinics website

281 Aliment Pharmacol Ther. 2001 Aug;15(8):1147-54
Anal sphincter biofeedback and pelvic floor exercises for faecal incontinence in
adults--a systematic review
Norton C, Kamm MA.
Physiology Unit, St Mark's Hospital, Harrow, UK.

282 https://en.wikipedia.org/wiki/Hydrotherapy
Wikipedia online encyclopedia: Hydrotherapy

283 Int J Clin Pract, March 2010, 64, 4, 429–431
Colonic irrigation: therapeutic claims by professional organisations, a review
E. Ernst -- Complementary Medicine, Peninsula Medical School, Exeter UK

284 https://www.jacuzzi.com/en-us/hot-tubs/blog/relaxation-and-other-
benefits-of-hydrotherapy
RELAXATION AND OTHER BENEFITS OF HYDROTHERAPY
Jaxuzzi Products website Jun 30, 2015

285 J Clin Periodontol. 1986 Mar;13(3):228-36.
The effects of a simplified oral hygiene regime plus supragingival irrigation with
chlorhexidine or metronidazole on chronic inflammatory periodontal disease.
Aziz-Gandour IA, Newman HN.

286   Vopr Kurortol Fizioter Lech Fiz Kult. 1989 Sep-Oct;(5):44-7.
[The action of massage on lymph formation and transport]. [Article in Russian]
Potapov IA, Abisheva TM.

287   Eur J Surg. 1992 Jun-Jul;158(6-7):347-50.
Comparison between sterile saline and tap water for the cleaning of acute traumatic soft tissue wounds.
Angerås MH1, Brandberg A, Falk A, Seeman T.
Department of Surgery, Medical Microbiology, University of Göteborg, Sweden.

288   YJFAS51411_proof 4 April 2013
Does Postoperative Showering or Bathing of a Surgical Site Increase the Incidence of Infection? A Systematic Review of the Literature
Paul Dayton, Mindi Feilmeier, Shelly Sedberry,
Podiatric Medicine and Surgery Residency, Trinity Regional Medical Center; IA

289   Techniques in Coloproctology January 2017, Volume 21, Issue 1, pp 1–4
Irrigation, lavage, colonic hydrotherapy - from beauty center to clinic
G. Bazzocchi
Neurogastroenterology and Intestinal Rehabilitation, Montecatone Rehabilitation Institute, University of Bologna, Italy

290   Techniques in Coloproctology August 2016, Volume 20, Issue 8, pp 551–557
Treatment of irritable bowel syndrome with a novel colonic irrigation system - a pilot study
H.-H. Hsu, W.-H. Leung
Division of Colorectal Surgery, Department of SurgeryMackay Memorial HospitalTaipei CityTaiwan

291   https://en.wikipedia.org/wiki/Islamic_toilet_etiquette
Wikipedia online encyclopedia: Wikipedia, "Islamic toilet etiquette"

292   http://mentalfloss.com/article/76994/6-practical-ways-romans-used-human-urine-and-feces-daily-life
6 Practical Ways Romans Used Human Urine and Feces in Daily Life
KRISTINA KILLGROVE
Mentalfloss website MARCH 14, 2016

293   http://www.dovetailinc.org/report_pdfs/2014/dovetailtreefree0714.pdf
TREE-FREE PAPER - A PATH TO SAVING TREES AND FORESTS
DR. JIM BOWYER, DR. JEFF HOWE, DR. ED PEPKE, etal
Dovetail Partners 8/19/2014

294   Am J Ind Med. 1991;20(6):769-74.
Mortality pattern among pulp and paper mill workers in Sweden: a case-referent study.
Wingren G1, Persson B, Thorén K, Axelson O.
Department of Occupational Medicine, University Hospital, Linköping, Sweden.

295   space & culture vol. 5 no. 4, november 2002 368-386
Flush With Success Bathing, Defecation, Worship, and Social Change in South India
Tulasi Srinivas -- Boston University

296   https://www.nytimes.com/2015/04/30/technology/personaltech
/electronic-bidet-toilet-seat-is-the-luxury-you-wont-want-to-live-without.html
Electronic Bidet Toilet Seat Is the Luxury You Won't Want to Live Without
Farhad Manjoo -- New York Times, Personal Tech GADGETWISE April 29, 2015

297   https://thoughtcatalog.com/james-b-barnes/2015/05/justbuttthings/
?utm_campaign=article&utm_source=thoughtcatalog&utm_term=james-b-
barnes&utm_medium=entry_related
25 Fun And Gross Things You Didn't Know About Your Butt
James B Barnes -- Thought Catalog website (2015)

298   http://laffgaff.com/funny-poop-jokes-and-puns/
LaffGaff website, home of fun and laughter
Funny Poop Jokes And Puns

299   Entry on my Facebook page from an old friend, David Gower

300   https://www.brondell.com/healthy-living-blog/returning-the-favor-how-
to-clean-a-bidet-toilet-seat-and-nozzle/
RETURNING THE FAVOR: HOW TO CLEAN A BIDET TOILET SEAT AND
NOZZLE
Brondell website sells bidets   Sept 25, 2018

301   https://www.wikihow.com/Clean-a-Bidet
How to Clean a Bidet   March 29, 2019
Co-authored by Michelle Driscoll
Wiki How To Do Anything website:

302   https://bidetking.com/blog/how-to-safely-clean-a-bidet-toilet-seat/
How to Safely Clean a Bidet Toilet Seat
Bidet King Website September 15, 2014

303   https://www.us.kohler.com/us/Care-&-Cleaning/article/CNT121300049.htm
[Bidet] Care and Cleaning
Kohler website

304   https://www.totousa.com/filemanager_uploads/product_assets/
D08886_C100_A100_OM_EN.pdf
Washlet A100 User's Manual: Maintainance
Toto USA website

305   https://www.medicalnewstoday.com/articles/17685.php
What's to know about dioxins
Christian Nordqvist   21 April 2017
Reviewed by Debra Rose Wilson, PhD, MSN, RN, IBCLC, AHN-BC, CHT
Medical News Today Website

306   http://www.poopiepoems.com/?offset=1404952560653
POOPIE POEMS, The Largest Collection of Poo Poetry on the web!

307   Environ Health Perspect 124:437–444; 2016
Bisphenol A, bisphenol S, and 4-hydroxyphenyl 4-isoprooxyphenylsulfone
(BPSIP) in urine and blood of cashiers.
Thayer KA, Taylor KW, Garantziotis S, etal

National Institute of Environmental Health Sciences, (NIEHS), Research Triangle Park, NC

308 https://www.reddit.com/r/educationalgifs/comments/aoslhl/ this_is_ how_ external_hemorrhoids_are_removed/
Reddit website - This is how External Hemorrhoids are removed!

309 Medica Innovatica, December 2013, Volume 2 - Issue 2
Current concept of pathophysiology and Biochemical factors involved in acute and chronic anal fissure
Amrut Dambal , Samata Padaki , B. Kusuma Kumari , etal
 Department of Biochemistry, Department of Physiology, Mallareddy Institute of Medical Sciences, Hyderabad, Andra Pradesh, India

310 https://cosmosmagazine.com/chemistry/the-world-is-running-out-of-phosphorus-and-that-s-a-really-bad-thing
The world is running out of phosphorus. And that's a really bad thing
Cosmos Magazine: The Science of Everything
Petr Kilian, Senior Lecturer, Chemistry,
University of St Andrews

311 http://design-ties.blogspot.com/2009/03/to-bidet-or-not-to-bidet.html
Design Ties Blog - MEADE DESIGN GROUP said...

312 Wikipedia - Toilet-related injuries and deaths citing
John Voelz, *King Me* (Littleton, CO 2010)

313 https://www.reddit.com/r/Frugal/comments/23gj8h/a_month_ago _i_bought_a_bidet_for_25_in_that_time/   - u/grouch1980
Reddit website

Photo Credits

I am most grateful for the many pictures graciously put into the public domain by individuals, particularly irom Wikipedia and Wikimedia. Several bidet retailers have also given permission to use graphics from their websites. A picture is truly worth a thousand words; this book is much better for their gracious support.

Cover Photo   Darling Classic Bidet (with horizontal nozzle) and matching toilet, courtesy Duravit Corp. Their website is www.duravit.us

Page   **Source**

Inside Title page -toto-washlet-s550e-installation – Toto Washlet TSB bidet (totousa.com)

1-sanicare100 handheld-Sanicare corp (sanicare.com)

3-A toilet and bidet at Shangri-La Barr Al Jissah Resort & Spa,Oman – Wikimedia – Aumars - GNU

3-Side view of a toilet seat bidet (TSB) with the seat open - Authors pic

4-Fauteuil_à_l'anglaise_et_bidet_au_XVIII_e_siècle – Wikipedia - Public Domain

5-Patent US07013502-20060321-D00006

6-Classic bidet-Basan1980 - German Wikipedia - Public Domain

6-Traditional French bidet beside toilet-Wikipedia-Lenilucho-GNU

6-Palma Vita bidet-Clos O Mat (closomat.co.uk)

6-Aerojet Shower Toilet - Clos-O-Mat Corp (closomat.co.uk)

7-Quoss premium bidet Q6000- Ksb1120-Wikimedia-GNU

7-My handheld bidet that I have used for years. Just a standard kitchen sink vegetable sprayer. Note wiping rag tucked below the toilet bowl - Author pic

7-   Not-PANASONIC-Portable-Washlet-Toilette-Bidet-Battery-Operated-Made-in-Japan

8-Classic bidet has the addition of a horizontal water jet with hot/cold faucets - Author pic

9-Darling classic bidet-Duravit Corp (www.duravit.us)

10-A 20th century standalone bidet-Lenilucho-Wikipedia-GNU

11- Wikimedia-Antekbojar (Poland)-PAŁAC PREZYDENCKI. ZABYTKOWA UBIKACJA-GNU.jpg

12-swash-s1000-bidet-toilet-seat-lifestyle-installed-shot1 (888-542-3355)

13-Otohime device in the ladies' toilet-Chris73-Wikipedia-GNU

14-Japanese bidet toilet in operation- Wikipedia - Chris73 - GNU

14-Magic Faucet parts illustration-Magic Faucet bidets (out of business)

16-Patent US06408451-20020625-D00002

16-line drawing of Bidematic bidet setup-Bidematic Corp (info@bidematic.com)

17-Washlet style toilet seat bidet (TSB) with side controls in showroom-Author pic

18-This is a wireless toilet control panel for a japanese toilet with 38 buttons. The model is a high-end model photographed in a Toto showroom-Wikimedia-Chris-GNU

19-Swash S-100 toilet seat bidet-Brondell Corp (brondell.com)

20-Another view of my personal handheld bidet. Note how it taps into the toilet bowl water feed-Author pic

21-Handheld bidet-Wikipedia-Sv7n-GNU

21-Patent US07096518-20060829-D00004

22-Plumbing setup for a BidBidet bb-200 bidet-this type of bidet uses external hot and cold water lines rather than an enclosed hot water heater-BioBidet Corp (biobidet.com)

23-HB-25 Handheld Bidet Shattaf with Adjustable Pressure Shut-off Valve-(bidet4me)

24-Multipurpose Handheld Fortable Bidet-Bidets2go Co. (bidets2go.com.au)

25-Handheld portable bidet-Porta-bidet Corp (porta-bidet.com)

25-Patent US20110016624A1-20110127-D00001

26-Cat on the bidet-Wikimedia-MisterDesgraciao-GNU

28-Squat toilet on the train with grab bar. White hose on bottom left is the vietnamese bidet-Brian Johnson & Dane Kantner-Wikimedia-GNU

28- The buttons on a Japanese bidet-style toilet to inject-stop the jet of water-Stefan Le Du from Nantes, France-Wikimedia-GNU

30-Patent - US20140101838A1-20140417-D00003-

33-Patent A US20140101838A1-20140417-D00005-A

34-Kindergarten-UDDT-Wikimedia-GNU

35-Musée_des_horreurs_24-Wikipedia-Coquin-GNU

37-Muslim Shattaf-Sv7n-Wikipedia-GNU-2

38-Wireless Bidet Control Panel-Chris-Wikipedia-GNU

39-ALBA-BALAMAND-WSF-01 WATER CLOSET FIXTURE–WISSAM SHEKHANI-Wikimedia-GNU

40-Patent A US20140101838A1-20140417-D00005

40-Patent US07954181-20110607-D00017

40-Patent A US20140101838A1-20140417-D00005

43-Patent- US20140101838A1-20140417-D00003

44-Patent US20110016624A1-20110127-D00001

46-Patent USRE039930-20071204-D00000

48-Toilet seat bidet (TSB). Front view with the toilet seat raised-The nozzle emerges from the middle of the crossing plate when in use-Author pic

49-Size and Space for Approach and Use in Bathroom-Udchula-Wikimedia-GNU

51-Toilets and bidet for sale!–Wikimedia-Tomer Gabel,Israel-Akihabara-GNU

53-Hyjet bidet-Xiamen Yixingda Plastic Co (Fujian, China)

55-A wireless battery operated toilet control panel for the Japanese toilet-Chris73-Wikimedia-GNU

56-Bidematic bidet in action!-Author pic

60-Patent US4391004-1-b

61- Modern classic bidet mounted on wall with toilet behind-Lazienka-Poland-Wikipedia-GNU

63-Installing the bidet with the toilet seat removed. The Bidematic unit is attached to the toilet by the bolt in the upper left corner. The toilet seat is about to be bolted on top of the BideMatic, holding everything in place. You can just see the handle that swings the Bidematic into action in the lower left-Author pic

68- Ancient toilet sticks from the Nara period-Chris73-Wikipedia-GNU

72-B-Werk Besseringen-LoKiLeCh-WIkimedia-GNU

74-Chart showing various options for toilet seat bidets-Ksb1120-Wikimedia-GNU-1-Quoss Bidet (quoss.co.kr)

74- Chart showing various options for toilet seat bidets-Ksb1120-Wikimedia-GNU-2-Quoss Bidet (quoss.co.kr)

75-Closeup of the water sprayer on the bottom of a French bidet. Note that there is not one big spray but a bunch of little sprays fairly concentrated-Author pic

82- Old style toilet, bidet and sink-Alcimar Luiz Callegari-Wikimedia-GNU

84-How to use a Panasonic portable bidet – courtesy of Factory Outlet (no longer sells bidets)

85-Illustration of nozzle use in gential wash - INAX Luscence Advanced Bidet Toilet - INAX (Japan)

85-Illustration of nozzle use in anal wash - INAX Luscence Advanced Bidet Toilet - INAX (Japan)

87-Bathroom in suite with traditional bidet at Semiramis InterContinental Hotel Cairo-Daniel Mayer-Wikimedia-GNU

91-BioBidet bb300h plumbing detail-Biobidet Corp (biobidet.com)

92-Plumbing illustration for installing a Daelim bidet (buybidet.com) – courtesy of Factory Outlet (no longer sells bidets)

92-Bidanit bidet installation pic – Bidanit (no longer in business)

92-Magic Faucet full system diagram-Magic Faucet bidet (no longer in business)

93-BioBidet bb300h plumbing detail-Biobidet Corp (biobidet.com)

93-plumbing setup illustraton – BioBidet Corp (biobidet.com)

93-plumbing illustration for installing Biffy Bidets (biffy.com)

95-106-Patent- US20140101838A1-20140417-D00003

97-Escape..A Very Rough Guide to Getting Away from it All blog-Vicki- catch-up-with-the-sun.blogspot.com

98-Pumping Sewage on Crops for Fertilizer – Source-Harper's Weekly, 1890, Photo IV.1 in The Search For The Ultimate Sink by Joel A. Tarr, The University of Akron Press, 1996.

98-Sewerage as a Beverage-Source-Plate 7 of Sewers-Ancient & Modern, by Cyrenus Wheeler, Jr. in the Collections of the Cayuga County Historical Society, 5 (1887).

102-Medieval tossing of shit – public domain

106-Traditional bidet-basan1980-Wikipedia-public domain

109-The Manufacture of Drain Pipe (Clay Pipe) The Manufacturer and Builder, April 1881, p. 82.

112-Palma vita–Clos O Mat (closomat.co.uk)

115-A line of toilet seat bidets (TSB) in a showroom-Author pic

121-Toilet paper 500x magnification–Qlav bidet (vulcanfire@att.net)

124-Patent EP0837193A2

128-Darling bidet display-Darling corp (info@us.duravit.com)

133-Patent US07096518-20060829-D00000b

135-A long line of toilet seat bidets (TSB) at a showroom-Author pic

139- toto-washlet-s550e-installation-Toto Corp (totousa.com)

139-105-Typical plumbing connection for cold water bidets. Note the T-connector in the middle taps into the toilet tank water supply and now supplies the bidet with water – Author pic

140-Bidematic Factory, Argentina-Bidematic bidets (info@bidematic.com)

142-Interior of the wheelchair-accessible toilet in a JR East E6 series Shinkansen train-掬茶-WIkimedia-GNU

142-Travel bidet How To Panasonic-courtesy of Factory Outlet (no longer sells bidets)

145-Antique bidet – Superco blog (discover.superco.net-what-is-a-bidet-bidet-antique)

152-Modern toilet seat bidet (TSB) in a showroom, with plumbing visible on the side-Author pic

188-My water supply setup for my handheld bidet. The big white hose at top right is the water feed to the toilet (going up), and a T-junction to tap water for the bidet is usually done where it connects with the water feed (lower right). My hardware guru Robert at my local hardware store Mendo-Mill found **a special junction** that allowed me to split-off water lines to two bidets (going left). It would have been difficult to fit all this additional hardware into the existing water line configuration. Author pic.

"Sanitation researchers often complain that the issues don't get the attention they deserve because shit is taboo, it is dirty and disgusting and no one wants to talk about it," explained Bell. "Except that everyone does. Once you start talking to people about toilets they won't shut up…It is a curious thing that on a personal level everyone wants to talk about toilets, but on a political level it's hard to get traction.[27]

A month ago, I bought a bidet for $25. In that time I have used less than one roll of toilet paper. There are a ton of bidets on Amazon for less than $100. I bought an Astor. It took 20 min. to install. Bidets are great for saving money, feeling cleaner, and preventing hemorrhoids. I highly recommend it.[313]

Appendices

How I Manage My Slow Reluctant Defecation with a Bidet

Danger: Using handheld bidets as described below can be dangerous and is strongly NOT recommended. That being said, knowing that the use of bidets is, and has been for a long time, used by at least thousands to directly induce defecation, this section is an attempt to defuse conflicting information with the best information I have, which is twenty years of my personal experience, which may not be your condition or experience. This book does contain everything known to peer-review science about bidets, but it is added to and mixed throughout with hearsay and weird opinions. **This book should be considered an exhortation to use bidets responsibly for their economy and cleanliness; compared to the excessive waste and un-cleanliness of TP culture.**

I am one of those unfortunate humans whose defecation is so slow that I would often lose circulation in my legs before I was "done" – I would be on the john so long that my legs and butt could barely work to get off the john. Not healthy. Worse still, I got so frustrated that I started pushing myself into hemorrhoids.

Do not consider anything in this book as medical advice; this book recommends that you do not do this method, certainly not without oversight of a medical professional.

In our clinic we find that people with all kinds of skin problems (i.e., acne, psoriasis, eczema, etc.) usually can benefit from a therapeutic course of colon irrigations. The skin is the largest excretory organ in the body. When the colon is sluggish or clogged up or there are a lot of toxins in the body, the skin may act as a major excretory organ. Unhealthy skin is usually a sign of an unhealthy colon and no amount of antibiotics, skin creams or medications will alleviate the problems until the cause of the problem is addressed... Almost every human ailment has been attributed to a malfunctioning colon (i.e., one that cannot perform its normal, regular and efficient functioning) - Donald J. Mantell, M.D.[277]

I can remember my very Scottish grandmother banging angrily on her outhouse door while I cowered inside. My mother was outside trying to mollify her, but granny was upset that I was using too much toilet paper while monopolizing her outhouse! As a child I was a problem pooper. I would camp out in our family bathroom for quite a while trying to poop. And when I finally did, I often had to do it all over again, maybe several times. All through life I have tried everything to speed up my pooping to no avail – until the bidet.

If you just want to help stimulate your defecation, I recommend you begin by purchasing a bidet with a good anal cleanse mode. This will both encourage a bowel movement and will wash you clean afterward. There are even bidets that advertise a strong "enema" mode. If this takes care of your eliminative needs then by all means get one of those bidets, they are a much cleaner and easier solution. I really do not recommend my method if at all avoidable. Even if you intend to use a handheld, you will not regret having a TSB bidet as well.

A high-pressure water jet flow is now provided by some of the manufacturers to aid defecation. It is considered that since the water pressures in these jets are higher than resting anal sphincter pressure water might penetrate into the rectum. By measuring increases in rectal temperature after applying warm water, we were able to confirm that this is the case. Accordingly, if water ingress exceeds this capacity, rectal pressures could elevate and promote defecation. We consider that the bidet defecatory function is poorer than a simple enema in terms of evoking anal sphincter contractions, although it is considered to be considerable more convenient by bidet users.[170]

[2016] Seventy-nine (230) individuals were using the warm-water washing toilet seat. There was no significant difference in age between the usage group and the non-use group. The purposes of use after defecation, for defecation induction, and after urination and for washing the vagina were 90.4, 41.3, and 40.4%, respectively. Regarding the kinds of washing, a strong tendency for the use of the anal washing function to induce defection and after defecation was observed, whereas a tendency was observed for the use of the bidet function after urination and for washing the vagina. Many individuals were using the washing function for the purpose of inducing defection and after urination.[206]

Many who are constipated need more internal pressure than others (which usually means higher rectal volumes) to get their bodies to defecate. Rectal contractions, anal relaxation, and a desire to defecate all require more pressure.[165,168] This has been covered in **Bowel Dysfunction: Constipation**.

How much more volume is needed to induce deification? In one study, fluid was introduced into the rectum to see how much displacement was needed to induce defecation. The results showed that 20-60 ml was enough to stimulate most constipated individuals (60 ml equals about 2 fluid ounces, 1/4 cup, or 4 tablespoons).[169] This is valuable to me, because it only takes a small amount of water to really stimulate my body and evacuation happens right away!

Why would anyone use a handheld bidet when many other effortless, automatic bidets are available? One factor is price, balancing a $15 handheld device against a $150+ for a basic TSB solution or $400 and up for a top-of-the-line bidet. Additionally handheld units are not very visible and take up little space.

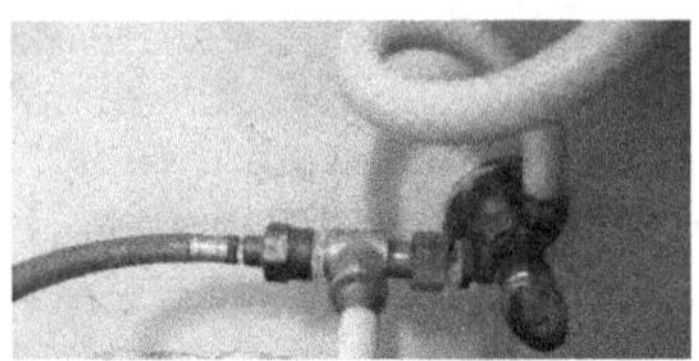

The big reason for me and probably most handheld users is the additional power, and the potential precision and accuracy of this cleaning experience (which puts responsibility on the operator every time). Handheld units can be much worse at washing when a beginner's hand can make a significant, disgusting mess by blasting feces all over the toilet area, while otherwise having no effect on their eliminative process. A practiced hand can apply the spray with surgical accuracy and utter cleanliness, and can certainly induce defecation within seconds in a completely gentle manner. Even those stiff constipated clay-like stools that will not fit through as constipated, can be softened and lubricated enough to be reformed into a shape that can be eliminated without pain or injury. The keys to using a handheld unit cleanly are appropriate water pressure, sensitivity and accuracy.

Before we go any further, there are two physical reasons why my method may not work for you: your water source is unsuitable, or your skin is too vulnerable.

Your water is too strong, its quality is unusable

Unlike my outer skin, my human rectum [which is also epitheilium, "skin"] has no ability to feel pain, heat, or other sensations, although it is quite sensitive to swelling from internal pressure.[166] So my first priority is to ensure that my water jet is not one single strong stream and that my water pressure is not too high or damaging. I must also be aware that any additives to my water supply will be absorbed by my rectum. It's a cost-benefit decision; you benefit by the water causing a bowel movement and cleaning out your rectum, the cost is a somewhat additional absorption of bad water things by your body each time you do this. Best to keep your business as short and your water as pure as possible.

People do not realize that our epithelium (outer skin, GI tract, lungs, etc) is highly absorptive. For example, the college prank of injecting alcohol directly into someone's colon can be fatal. Alcohol absorbed directly through your epitheilium (your skin, which includes the lining of your colon), bypasses the liver, which is your body's main detoxification organ. Without this processing of alcohol by the liver you body can receive a smaller fatal amount of alcohol much easier. I guess you can still drink yourself to death directly, but it tends to be much harder to do and takes longer. This is just a reminder that whatever you put in your rectum/colon (either way) is absorbed directly into your body.

Municipal water may be too dangerous to inject into your colon. Municipal water is universally treated with some form of chlorine, plus perhaps other unspecified additives. My water supply is from a natural spring. It is not treated in any way, certainly not any form of chlorine which I consider toxic. My colon is dedicated to removing any water for later excretion as urine, which means any toxins in my water are absorbed from my GI tract (usually over days) into my system. I do not have to balance an added exposure to chlorine (and other additives) because my water is actually quite pure except for an excess of acidity.

First and foremost: and already frequently mentioned, the shape of my water jet is very important; My sprayer has about 32 little jets which deliver a very useful spray for my needs. Page 20 has a good illustration. This is very important: to diffuse the force of water while still keeping it focused enough to overcome my anus. It is crucial for me to have a force that works but is kind to my skin.

Second: I keep the water pressure of my bidet at relatively low pressures of 15-40 psi. Most municipal water supplies run on high pressures of 80-100+ pounds per square inch pressure. I would say 15 psi would be a good place to start.

Water Spray Questionable With Injured Skin

Colorectal surgeons have been reluctant to use electronic bidets because the high force of water from commercially used electronic bidets may harm the anus.[20,106] On the other side many users have eagerly embraced a more concentrated higher-pressure spray, when available, for the express purpose of inducing defecation.[130] Water pressure and spray pattern can be fully adjustable with many modern TSB bidets.

It is physically dangerous to direct any strong water stream at any rectum or perianal area that has any significant breaks, weaknesses, or defects. If you have anal fissures, popped hemorrhoids, particularly weak skin, or anything like that, applying any force of water into your rectum could be dangerous and could be further injuring. If you resemble this, I strongly recommend that you do not follow my methods described here, and discuss this with a qualified health professional before using any bidet.

The benefits of a simple water spray on irritated or damaged skin have been discussed in previous sections[93-6] but you must also be very careful with injured skin, especially in the perianal area. If you must begin any cleansing in your perianal region, please at least begin at very low water pressure.

As women age, the lining of the vaginal and bladder skin becomes thin and more easily irritated, requiring more gentle care. This may predispose a woman to bladder and vaginal infections. As men age they are susceptible to similar infections. The bidet is excellent for reducing the likelihood of bacteria being inadvertently introduced into these sensitive areas.[102,191]

An anal fissure is a break or tear in the skin of the anal canal. Anal fissures may be noticed by bright red anal bleeding on toilet paper and undergarments, or sometimes in the toilet. If acute they are painful after defecation. **Most anal fissures are caused by stretching of the anal**

mucosa [epithelium] beyond its capability. Superficial or shallow anal fissures look much like a paper cut, and may be hard to detect upon visual inspection, they will generally self-heal within a couple of weeks.[2]

How I Do It

For years I was satisfied with just using my bidet to wash off after defecation. Then, despite this I developed a case of external hemorrhoids - two skin bubbles almost blocking my anus. Worse, they wouldn't go away. In the past, applying Preparation H would eventually shrink them, but not this time. I applied so much Preparation H I was sliding around in my pants, but my hemorrhoids were not getting better. Once these enlarged veins have been weakened, all it takes is a little push to re-inflate my hemorrhoids (or to make them worse), and pushing was both my modus operandi and my habit.

I get hemorrhoids from being impatient. Being at work, in a hurry, and frustrated at the usual long slow progress of my elimination causes me to start straining to defecate. Forcing bowel movements, day after day, eventually weakens certain veins and causes hemorrhoids. After nearly a month of having a greasy butt with nothing to show for it, it occurred to me that my bidet might be of help. What a revelation! Directly applied to my anus it really helps to have an effortless bowel movement! Effortless is salvation from hemorrhoids.

First of all, it is about relaxation, something in short supply in our world. I can shoot water directly at my anus all day and if my sphincter does not relax, nothing is going to happen. It can and will tighten up, in my case almost always after my first and main defecation. You are going to have to relax into using a handheld, and relax your attitude towards your body and particularly towards your reluctant bottom. It will come out if you coax it out gently, over time.

Unlike your skin, the rectum has no ability to feel pain, heat, or other sensations, but is quite sensitive to swelling from internal pressure.[166]

My sphincter at first resisted this new sensation of water attacking it from outside; nevertheless over time benefiting from this water pressure it has generally relaxed its attitude and actions (pun). Over time it has become much easier to relax and allow my rectum to be opened by my bidet's water pressure.

Sitting on my toilet, I snake my handheld between my legs so that it is positioned under my anus pointing up. Keep the spray head an inch or two away with some short initial squirts. After applying a small amount of spray to wash off anything hanging onto my anus or in my perianal area, then

I position the spray head into direct contact directly over my anus, and held with some nominal pressure against it forming a sort of seal.

Water pressure builds up until it overcomes my sphincter's resistance, then leaks past my stools lubricating them on the way, and continues to fill my rectum until it reaches another stool impasse and pressure builds up. As soon as my body signals significant pressure has built up, I stop and immediately remove the spray head. Do not ever push that sense of pressure from your colon, treat it as a cry for help, always stop as soon as you can feel it. It only takes seconds for my body to react and eliminate. I usually have to repeat this 2-3 times to be sure I am "done".

Strangely, at times, even after years of using my handheld bidet, it is hard to find my anus! But it is imperative to have its head centered and in close contact for me to administer enough water pressure to blow past my stools, lubricating them all around as they pass; then accumulating enough water above my stools to provide just enough pressure on top to motivate defecation.

To relieve hemorrhoids, constipation, or to help anyone who has a long, hard time inducing a bowel movement, defecation must somehow be induced without strain or forcing. This bidet hydro-massage can ease those tight, retentive anuses like mine that specialize in reluctant, slow elimination that can lead to hemorrhoids. We have previously explored how hydro-massage relaxes and stimulates the sphincter muscles of the anus.

In a study of females with obstructed defecation, 76 per cent stated they applied physical pressure in the anal region, and this stimulated their process of elimination. The researchers agreed that external pressure increased rectal tone and aided the women's efforts.[74]

This morning I was inexplicably constipated. I could feel a substantial mass of stool blocking any elimination like a big seal. My procedure at first was no different: shoot water up my rectum to lubricate the obstinate stool, leaving some water up top as well to stimulate. The water involved softened the constipated stool, allowing me to use my rectal muscles to squeeze it into a narrower shape (like molding clay) that could then pass without difficulty.

On the other hand diarrhea is more complicated with much more mess. I rarely get diarrhea but it does happen. Pretty much the only time I soil my drying rag is when I have diarrhea – its mess is so sneaky! Flushing diarrhea out of my rectum has a couple of benefits for me: all my watery shit has been removed from my immediate colon then buys me a little rest time before leaking resumes; cleaning out the rectum with clean water can sometimes be the sole solution for my diarrhea.

After First Defecation

Especially if I have hemorrhoids, applying the water massage several more times encourages any remaining bowel movement to continue. Irrigating and massaging my anus also gives me a better feel for whether I am really done - it kind of "calls the question".

It may be that you do not need help in initiating a bowel movement, but you may need help in finishing it. Research and surveys of people who suffer from constipation or diarrhea, find that all of them, old people and young, complain about feelings of incompletion, of feeling they still have to go.[144,176]

I am rarely done with one bowel movement, even with the help of my bidet. My general need is to repeat this process, to inject water 2-3 times more to completely clear my colon. As long as something comes out, I keep spraying, and each time there is defecation there is room for more water to go deeper. Sometimes I shit once and my rectum closes up and that is it for my uncertain rectum. You develop a sensitivity to where your rectum is at.

Despite all of that I will at times still have what I call a "hanging chad" of stool, a small stool that hasn't come out but hangs back just inside my rectum. As I stand up and re-clothe, and perhaps take a step or two all-of-a-sudden I need to shit again. I can ignore it but it will bother me all day. Re-inducing defecation often brings out a lot more stool, rather than just this irritating little fragment. Every once and a while I have to do another bowel movement a third time or a fourth.

Other studies of constipation and obstructed defecation have found that biofeedback therapy works very well. Biofeedback usually consists of techniques to induce relaxation of muscles that control elimination, and subsequently retraining these muscles and nerves. After biofeedback therapy, symptomatic improvement has been reported in 70 to 80% of patients with either incontinence or obstructive defecation. Recent studies also shown objective improvement in anorectal function.[75] Read more in the section on **Hydo-Massage**.

The results show that all these children were successfully conditioned to relax their anal sphincter during defecation. This therapy improved their bowel habits and relieved them from constipation and soiling... Biofeedback therapy seems to be the appropriate treatment in such cases.[76]

When rising from my toilet these days I either have a true and real sense of "being done", or those few times when I do have lingering incompleteness, I know I am at least clean all over outside and usually at least a few inches inside.

I personally have found that using my handheld bidet to relax and induce elimination - has over time some-how retrained my body towards generally faster and easier "natural" bowel movements. When my bidet is not available for stimulation (usually only when traveling) my elimination has nevertheless become more easy and natural than my previous travel difficulties pre-bidet. Traveling, I will start the first days of my travel using laxative tea but after that my bowel movements are pretty normal – still delicate but relatively normal.

Clean Up After

When using a handheld bidet it is important to do a quick visual inspection of the toilet seat, top and bottom, and toilet bowl after every defecation. It can be fast but should be observant. Regular bidets do not need anywhere near the same care and caution as handhelds. My shit often first comes out as a lump that splashes into the toilet water; things like that need to be followed up. Your handheld bidet can be a main agency of cleaning, with care (again) it can give most everything a power wash. My handheld bidet is also useful for cleaning our toilet bowl, with full pressure it can sometimes unclog our sewer line (usually caused by my wife's TP use), and can even reach into our shower stall for some additional washing. Diapers, washcloths, underpants that have been significantly soiled, or any other soiled garments, can be washed relatively clean by my bidet's spray as well.

My original goal - a cleaner derriere without wasting toilet paper - is still the most satisfying. While I occasionally use toilet paper for other cleaning purposes, it is never used for anal cleaning anymore unless I am traveling.

Deep Breathing

At times deep breathing can really help my defecation. Breathing in and out really deep massages and squeezes my digestive residue down my colon. This is very useful when I do not have a bidet. Twenty deep breaths can often induce defecation, and if it does not, it at least compacts things and makes elimination easier and faster. Singing exercises often encourage deep breathing as well.

Deep breathing can be accomplished sitting down in a meditative posture such as lotus posture, or sitting on a chair or standing up with your spine held straight. First check your posture. The spine should be straight, the head erect, hands on knees, mouth closed. Now concentrate on the pharyngeal space at the back wall of your mouth and, slightly contracting its muscles, begin to draw in the air through that space as if you were using a suction pump. Do it slowly and steadily, letting the pumping sound be clearly heard. Don't use the nostrils; remember that they remain inactive during the entire respiration process. When inhaling let your ribs expand sideways like an accordion-beginning with the lower ones, of course. Remember the chest and shoulders should remain motionless.

The entire inhalation should be done gently and effortlessly. When it has been completed pause for a second or two, holding the breath. Then slowly begin breathing out. The exhalation is usually not as passive as the inhalation. You use a slight, a very slight, pressure to push the air out-although it feels as though you pressed it against the throat like a hydraulic press. The upper ribs are now contracted first, the nostrils remain inactive and the chest and shoulders motionless. At the end of the exhalation, pull in the stomach a little so as to push out all the air.[79]

Anatomically, the best position to defecate is from a deep crouch but our toilets are not designed to allow this. Most of us physically couldn't crouch that deep or long enough to complete the act anyhow. I find the stimulation that the bidet spray provides can overcome a lot of this postural disadvantage.

Yoga breathing significantly helps my elimination. Yoga uses deep breaths as an effective way to stretch abdominal muscles and gain muscle tone. Deep breathing is also used in singing classes to improve projection. It is also effective as massaging and encouraging transit of my defecation down my colon. Taking deep breaths occupies more space inside, slightly compressing and exercising my other organs, especially my bladder and colon. This stimulates these organs into action. This is a natural, non-straining way to move things along, basically the antithesis of trying to "push" my stools out and causing hemorrhoids.

I am not "pushing" like I'm trying to fart and thus causing hemorrhoids. Inhaling all that air causes body organs to move around a bit from the stomach to the anus. rather I am squeezing my colon like a tube of toothpaste, or rolling my belly like a belly dancer, keeping the main stress away from my colon. Walking and exercise of course accomplishes the same thing, and deep breathing is sort of pretending that you are working hard.

I might try up to 20 deep breaths, and if there are not any encouraging signs from my anus, then I will give up and employ my bidet. In any case such breathing helps to compact my stools which in this case is good. Of course a certain amount of exercise will also achieve this. My retired life is very sedentary (little physical encouragement to move things along) and I would be in trouble but for my bidet.

"For the first time, researchers have found a person in the United States carrying bacteria resistant to antibiotics of last resort, an alarming development that the top U.S. public health official says could mean "the end of the road" for antibiotics. It's the first time this colistin-resistant strain has been found in a person in the United States. In November, public health officials worldwide reacted with alarm when Chinese and British researchers reported finding the colistin-resistant strain in pigs and raw pork and in a small number of people in China. The deadly strain was later discovered in Europe and elsewhere. "It basically shows us that the end of the road isn't very far away for antibiotics — that we may be in a situation where we have patients in our intensive care units, or patients getting urinary-tract infections for which we do not have antibiotics." CDC Director Tom Frieden said in an interview. [The Washington Post, May 27,2016]. **See my ad for the world's most powerful herbal antibiotic and antifungal on the last page of this book.**

How I Wipe My Arse   *by Brian Ferri-Taylor*

My spouse has made ass wipes from an old white towel. They are terry cloth about 8 X 8" square and hemmed on all sides. A softer, yet absorbent, material might be nice. A regular washcloth is rather large for the purpose and a handkerchief is too thin. White is important because I will re-use a cloth until some/any "color" shows. Clean cloths are stored in a drawer easily accessible while seated on the bidet. When done, I start the water wash at a low stream intensity and increase it to high. I relax my anus and give myself a mini enema, turn the water off and hold for several seconds. I angle my bum hole forward a bit by rocking my pelvis back. I want the final emptying to be directed into the water, not to the back sides of the bowl. Done with that, I turn the water back on and wiggle my bum around a little to get at all the spots that need cleaning. I now have water dripping from my bum. I obtain a wipe and position it next to my hip in preparation for standing. As I start to rise, I quickly move the cloth to catch any drip and then wipe from a slight squat. I then place the cloth draped over the shower door to dry. The trick here is to remember to fetch the used cloth the next time on my way to the toilet. I have a one gallon plastic milk jug filled with bleach water (1/2 cup 8.25% bleach/gallon of water) stored under the sink. A soiled towel usually shows just a little color and next to never any solids. I place the soiled towel, opened and flat, in the sink. I pour a small amount of bleach water onto the spot. I do not pre- or post- rinse. I fold the spot into the cloth and rub until it is gone. I then place the cloth into a bucket (also under the sink). On wash day we are handling, usually dry, visually clean, bleached cloths. I wash my hands and flush the toilet. Two notes of caution: (1) a bleached wipe, even dry, will ruin colored clothes included in the wash; (2) My spouse does not use the BioBidet because the water is cold and she fears the spray is too much back-to-front and increases the risk of vaginitis.

BUENOS AIRES, BIDET MECCA

by Jorge Rebagliati (Quest Bidets: questgreensolutions.com)

It is well known that the bidet was conceived in France in the first half of the 18th century (1700s) and then enjoyed great design and engineering improvements in England during the second half of the 19th century and beginning of the 20th. What is not well known is that the use of bidets flourished in the 20th century in Buenos Aires, the "Paris of South America", probably more than anywhere else in the world.

Between 1880 and 1930, the inhabitants of the then very prosperous Buenos Aires, known as "porteños" (people of the port) were inspired by the European

culture in all ways, following very attentively all the trends that came from that part of the world.

With the discoveries by the French biologist and chemist Louis Pasteur, about the existence of microbes and their capability to cause illness in the human body, washing with water became an essential component of health practices in Europe towards the end of the 19th century. This new hygienic movement took root quickly and deeply in Buenos Aires, eliciting massive changes to personal hygiene practices and to the potable water and sewage services.

Washing the body with clean water became a common and desirable practice of the porteños, associated with the fulfillment of a social code that even had connotations of moral virtue. This change even caused complaints by the Bureau of Health Works, when it could not keep up with the demand for potable water during the summer of 1900 because "the whole Buenos Aires was bathing".

Buenos Aires embarked on a massive renovation that, by 1896, had 22,000 buildings connected to the sewage network. Most of the city was connected to it during the first two decades of the 20th century. The potable water pipe network also grew by leaps and bounds, achieving the supply of the total population by 1925.

Together with the evolution of the sewage and potable water networks came the evolution of the bathrooms. Bathtubs, showers, lavatories and bidets, mainly made in England, were avidly bought by the porteños as their residences were connected to the networks.

The latest advancements in bathroom fixtures came quickly to Buenos Aires, including, as early as 1901, bidets with hot and cold water and ascending (vertical) spray and a bidet apparatus with a movable metal spray wand that allowed incorporating the function of a bidet to a toilet.

Breaking with old moral prejudices and embracing the new principles of personal hygiene, the inhabitants of Buenos Aires adopted the bidet more and more as a permanent feature of the bathroom. The initial moderate acceptance of the bidet that lasted into the 20's, turned, soon after, into widespread acceptance and the bidet became a common and indispensable fixture of the bathrooms in Buenos Aires and the rest of the country. Buenos Aires became a leader in the use of the bidet, surpassing its original suppliers, England, France and the United States of America.

Now, in the 21st century, Buenos Aires continues to feature bidets or bidet systems, such as the Argentinean-made Bidematic, in most bathrooms. Its importance is reflected in the value of real estate, since a property with bathrooms that have no bidets or hook ups for bidet systems command lower prices in the market. To a porteño and to most Argentineans, daily personal hygiene without a bidet is simply unacceptable.

"I want to thank Jorge Rebagliati for his help in bringing my book to the public, and for his original support in offering *The Bidet* for sale. He shows rare courage and vision is his efforts to make bidets available and affordable to everyone in America." – Bill Bruneau, author of **The Bidet**

About the Author

Walked away from two degrees and a teaching credential at Cal Berkeley in the late 60s. Spent time in the Haight-Ashbury. Spent some time on the margins of society - until I became a father. That changed everything. Both my son and step-daughter eventually graduated from Stanford University.

For better or worse, I am one of the people who brought personal computers into being. I am a "76er" – anyone involved before 1976 was a genuine pioneer. I worked for the People's Computer Company of digital legend, as well as running database marketing for the very first Computer Faires. Once personal computing stopped being a crusade and became industry I lost interest and became a gardener of sorts. Having a computer background was very helpful when starting a seed company in the 1980s.

Around 1990 I created a laminated poster, **The Vegetable Gardener's Guide** (in its third printing), that has been a perennial favorite of master gardeners – they are grateful to have all the essential questions beginners ask right there on the wall in a sturdy water-resistant poster.

Publishing The Bidet

In 2004 I decided to put my enthusiasm for the French bidet into the first edition of this book. This book turned out to be the first book on the topic, ever! Could not find anything in print. There was nothing in the Library of Congress at the time except a note by President Thomas Jefferson on the bidet as a result of his visit to Paris in the 1700s. What a treat to write the first book on anything in 2004! I covered everything known at the time, and went beyond by adding information from other knowledge bases, resulting in a book whose information is still very complete and current today.

The Bidet immediately became the reference on the subject. It was commonly known in the industry as the "bidet bible", because it included every thing known about the bidet, and more.

Unpublished authors in 2004 had few options for publication. I ended up physically making every book, binding each one, and selling them on Amazon on consignment. Create Space publishing did not exist. So I printed pages through a cheap home printer, punched the spiral binding and bound the book.

I soon grew tired of physically producing books for a significant loss of time and materials and stopped publication. Nevertheless used copies (when available) were selling for $30. It is interesting how many thousand times it has been pirated on the web over those years! People really wanted this little book!

Bountiful Gardens

I have been in technology most of my adult life. My wife and I started Bountiful Gardens Seeds in 1982, which is part of Ecology Action of the Midpeninsula, an organization that has been desperately trying to save the world's soil for the last 45 years, while refining a farming method (biointensive) that actually creates soil while being very productive. I brought an immediate benefit by introducing computers and digital technology into EA and BG early on.

We started Bountiful Gardens because heirloom, open-pollinated seeds were hard to come by in the 1980s, and disappearing. At the time it was not certain that these heirloom seeds would continue to be available to the general public. We offered a considerable number of varieties that otherwise would not have been available, perhaps forever. For years I selected many of the varieties we carried in our catalog, which was not unlike being an Indiana Jones of the plant world.

I consider myself a personal herbalist. I do not have the intimate, extensive knowledge of hundreds of herbs that a professional herbalist would know, but rather I know very well the few plants that I need, seeking only my health, and the health of my family.

Genus Sida

Medicinal herbs and preventative medicine have been at the core of my family's health for at least 50 years. I know the plants I use very well, and when I discover a new one that is as good as Sida is, I am completely on board right away, and want to know everything about it. The next step is a thorough and intensive research into its known benefits. So for several years I intensely scoured the internet for peer-review research on Sida, and in particular studies on Sida acuta, the species that I use. The results have exceeded my wildest expectations.

I have since published two books on genus Sida that are available on Amazon.com:

Sida acuta, Sida cordifolia, Sida rhombifolia, Etc. Everything Science and Tradition Knows About the World's Best Herbal Antibiotics, Used by Millions of People Every Day, Top Ayurvedic Herbs, Protein-Rich Survival Plants, Superior Fiber, Grow Them with Your Tomatoes (563 pp, 809 citations, $30.00)

I call this the physician's desk reference to genus Sida, the most potent herbal medicinal in the world but completely unknown to Western herbals. Everything known about Sida's medicinal properties, which are immense (bbruneau.com

A User's Guide to Sida acuta, Sida cordifolia, and Sida rhombifolia:: How to Grow, Harvest, and Make the World's Best Herbal Antibiotics, Protein-Rich, Used by Millions, Grow Them Like Tomatoes (48 pp, $6.00 paper, $4.49 Kindle)

This book is for everyone else. A basic guide to selecting, planting, growing, harvesting, and making essential medicals from your crop. This is the result of my eight years of growing and processing Sida for my personal health.

It is hard for a generation raised on pharmaceutical antibiotics to understand herbal anti-pathogens (Sida is antibiotic, antifungal, anti-protozoa, anti-malarial, etc. With pharma we have to be careful not to overuse (although we do this hugely!). With herbal antipathogens there is no antibioitic resistance, basically the bugs never figure it out. Sida never interferes with pharma products, actually it augments the positive effects of pharma antibioitics and antifungals, and occasionally outperforms them in its native form. Generally if a Sida dose doesn't work, most herbalists who know Sida say to simply increase the dose.

Praise for The Bidet (first edition)

http://englishdictionary.education/en/bidet
English dictionary (A powerful English dictionary online with many examples of use: definitions, synonyms, translations, related news and books)
The Bidet: Everything There is to Know from the First and ...
This is the only complete and impartial source of bidet information. This book has interesting history, drama, suspense, some real eye-opening facts, and is pretty good reading for a reference book.

Library of Online Book Shopping http://1lg09.hostfree.pw/
Ronald G. Rubin   4.9 out of 5 stars.
"First, it's important to say this is not only a great little book, but it is a primer for our culture to shift into the 21st century... This book received significant support from the bidet industry while it was being written, but is an independent work that surveys the industry as a whole. This book presents and documents the medical literature that largely supports the many health benefits that bidet users claim."

Librabook website   http://librarbook.com/
Rating: 4.6/5 from 1158 votes.
Australian Bidet - the largest supplier of Bidets, Electronic Bidet Seats, Integrated Toilet Bidets, Non-Electric Bidet Seats, Bidet Attachments and Personal Hygiene products for Australia, New Zealand and South-east Asia.
"Known in the bidet industry as 'The Bidet Bible', this book will save you many times its price while improving your health and personal comfort. The Bidet contains everything known about the bidet."

http://jscms.jrn.columbia.edu/cns/2007-04-10/vinograd-bidets.html
Columbia News Service » Apr 10, 2007
Bringing in the bidets   By Cassandra Vinograd
But more and more Americans are installing combination bidet toilets that experts say are more sanitary and also add a touch of luxury.
"It's starting to manifest at the upper level that oftentimes determines taste and acceptance in this country," said William Bruneau, who wrote "The Bidet Book," a 90-page guide often referred to as the bible of the bidet industry.

Library Thing Review - A community of 2,100,000 book lovers.

Toby Marotta, May 12, 2011
This unprecedented American introduction to bidet use is a self-published paperback composed and periodically updated by Bill Bruneau. Bill is a self-educated home ecologist based in Northern Californian. He was horrified to discover that Americans tend to know little or nothing about modes of intimate cleansing people elsewhere in the world believe essential. So he made himself an expert on bidets and then wrote and self-published this unique little booklet about the benefits of equipping one's bathroom with some kind of device for intimate washing -- anything from a traditional European-style bowl bidet to a mobile sprayer attachment. "This is the only complete and impartial source of bidet information. This book has interesting history, drama, suspense, some real eye-opening facts, and is pretty good reading for a reference book."

http://jscms.jrn.columbia.edu/cns/2007-04-10/vinograd-bidets.html
Columbia News Service » Apr 10, 2007
Bringing in the bidets   By Cassandra Vinograd
But more and more Americans are installing combination bidet toilets that experts say are more sanitary and also add a touch of luxury.
"It's starting to manifest at the upper level that oftentimes determines taste and acceptance in this country," said William Bruneau, who wrote "The Bidet Book," a 90-page guide often referred to as the bible of the bidet industry.

http://www.growbiointensive.org/news-0508-pubs.htm
Ecology Action Website, August 2005 newsletter, "Publications"
The Bidet by William Bruneau (Self-published: publish@bbruneau.com, www.bbruneau.com; 2004; $7.95) is a full coverage of this little-known subject. The author has obviously done his research. He discusses different kinds and types of bidets and includes a comprehensive list of manufacturers and the features of their product, as well as listing retailers with their phone number and/or website. All of the many quotations within the text have citations. Bruneau also talks about the benefits of using a bidet, including health benefits. The body's natural functions are described in natural language, with much of this coming from the author's own experience. This is a good book for anyone who has thought about adding a bidet to their bathroom or for anyone interested in the subject.

https://www.treehugger.com/bathroom-design/bidets-eliminate-toilet-paper-increase-your-hygiene.html
Treehugger website, "Driving Green since 2004"
"Bidets: Eliminate Toilet Paper, Increase Your Hygiene"
Justin Thomas
(In conclusion) This book is a good source of information on bidets: Everything There Is To Know, From The First and Only Book On The Bidet. The book discusses the different models of bidets, the health aspects and ecological benefits.

http://australianbidet.com.au/publications.html

The Bidet: Everything there is to know, from the first and only book on The Bidet; The topic no one talks about, the device that can save your life - By William Bruneau

The first book ever on the bidet! Don't laugh or be embarrassed - the right bidet can be an incredibly effective tool for personal cleanliness, and this book explains everything! Known in the bidet industry as "The Bidet Bible", this book will save you many times its price while improving your health and personal comfort. The Bidet contains everything known about the bidet. This book exhaustively covers the subject. It delineates the many benefits that bidets offer: sheer comfort, personal cleanliness, perianal health, good ecology, and superior economy. The Bidet demystifies and introduces the reader to every type, every use, and every aspect of the various forms of the bidet. Everything known about the bidet is covered in an impartial consumer reports format.

The Sunday Times Sri Lanka
http://www.sundaytimes.lk/080706/Mirror/mirror0010.html
In defense of the hand-held hygiene gun!
By Rukshani Weerasooriya
"An obviously bored and very creative man. William Bruneau actually took the time to write The Bidet Book which is a 90 page guide on everything you ever wanted to know about your bidet. This book is often referred to as the Bible of the bidet industry. As fascinating a fact that this may be, I have spent many lonely moments of my day wondering how in the world a person could write 90 whole pages on the bidet."

"I have read with great interest the copy of "The Bidet" you kindly mailed me. You boldly deal with this subject which seems to be the victim of a long-standing conspiracy. You have covered all the different aspects of the bidet that need to be known by the consumer... Your work will be very helpful to wake up Americans to the reality of the bidet." – Jorge Rebagliati, Bidematic Bidet System

"I read the book cover to cover and found it very accurate, informative and good reading. "I am very interested in your book. I chose marketing this product because I truly believe in it. I have three units in my home, two at my office, one in my motor home and on my boat. I potty trained my kids on it and they refuse to sit on a cold seat."" Keith Chamblin, Hygiene For Health (perhaps the most knowledgeable bidet marketer in the U.S.)

"Thank you very much for your book. I received it before Christmas and already read several times... Basically you book is a very good sales weapon, with nice information..." – Mihail Lisu, Clean O Seat

"It's a great book! I enjoyed it a lot. Used it to help me update our website. I showed it to our owner, who is Taiwanese, and who has used a bidet all his life. He liked the book." – Marc Wallin, Feel Fresh Bidet

"As far as I can see, the book is a comprehensive bidet-bible of sorts (with an impressive circulation rate). Personally, I love the no-holds-barred attitude towards both subject matter and um...vocabulary". – Julie Geoghan, Duravit Corp.

Disclaimer (continued)

This disclaimer covers all material information of all types and forms in this book. The information contained in this book is in summary form only and is intended to provide broad consumer understanding and knowledge of the topics covered. **Text and information is not intended to diagnose, treat, cure or prevent any disease conditional or malady.** No warranty is made or given that any information in this book is complete and/or accurate, and no warranty is given on the accuracy or correctness of any of the material that is hereby published.

The information contained in this book is not intended to be a substitute for professional advice. Any user should always seek the advice of a professional prior to commencing to use any new device, supplement, or new treatment for any of the conditions diseases or maladies mentioned in this book. Information obtained by using this book is probably not exhaustive and should not be considered sufficient to act upon. **This book does not recommend any purchase of equipment, any course of construction or of repair, or self management of health problems beyond the recreational use of the bidet.** Advice furnished by a qualified physician, pharmacist, or other health care provider should never be disregarded, nor should any delay occur in seeking competent and qualified advice as a consequence of anything contained in this book.

Neither the writer nor the publisher accepts any responsibility for the accuracy of the information in this book nor the consequences arising from the application, use, or misuse of any of the information contained herein, including any injury and/or damage to any person or property as a matter of product liability, negligence, or otherwise.

Information in this book has come from a number of websites which do not warrant the accuracy or correctness of the information therein. The names of all devices and companies in this book are under the protection of trademark or copyright. No warranty, expressed or implied, is made in regard to the contents of this material or any of the devices described therein. This material is not intended as a guide to construction, installation, personal treatment, self-medication, nor any other action.

The writer and publisher of this book are no more responsible for the information contained herein, than is the custodian of information contained in a public library, in that **this book provides a convenient source of information collation, and no more**. Be advised that all information in this book has no warranty whatsoever. The reader takes full and total responsibility for what they do with the information in this book, and any resulting outcomes from subsequent actions.

The use of trade, firm, or corporation names in this book is for the information and convenience of the reader; this does not constitute an official endorsement or approval by the author of any product or service to the exclusion of others that may be available.

Use of this book gives no permission or legal right to use the trademarked or copyrighted material therein. With respect to any third party products, services, information, or data described in this book, any guarantees, representations, or warrantees are provided solely by the third party provider, and not by the author, publisher, or any other contributor.

The Boring Legal Stuff: This book is not designed to, and does not, provide medical advice. All content ("content"), including text, graphics, images and information available on or through this book are for general informational purposes only. The content is not intended to be a substitute for professional medical advice, diagnosis or treatment. Never disregard professional medical advice, or delay in seeking it, because of something you have read in this book. Never rely on information in this book in place of seeking professional medical advice.

For the first time, researchers have found a person in the United States carrying bacteria resistant to antibiotics of last resort, an alarming development that the top U.S. public health official says could mean "the end of the road" for antibiotics. It's the first time this colistin-resistant strain has been found in a person in the United States. In November, public health officials worldwide reacted with alarm when Chinese and British researchers reported finding the colistin-resistant strain in pigs and raw pork and in a small number of people in China. The deadly strain was later discovered in Europe and elsewhere. "It basically shows us that the end of the road isn't very far away for antibiotics — that we may be in a situation where we have patients in our intensive care units, or patients getting urinary-tract infections for which we do not have antibiotics." CDC Director Tom Frieden said in an interview. [The Washington Post, May 27, 2016]

This book can save your life

Sida acuta, Sida cordifolia, Sida rhombifolia, Etc: Everything Science and Tradition Knows About the World's Best Herbal Antibiotics, Used by Millions of People Every Day, Top Ayurvedic Herbs, Protein-Rich Survival Plants, Superior Fiber, Grow Them with Your Tomatoes   Published Januuary 2018 567 pages   809 citations   Price $29.45

- Sidas are consumed by millions of people every day all over the world for a wide array of health problems, and people have been healing themselves with Sidas for thousands of years.
- Sidas control or kill 27 pathogenic bacteria, including many resistant strains, including MRSA.
- Sidas have good effect against malaria and other parasites.
- Sidas have tested well against 16 different pathogenic fungi, including 15 strains of candida.
- Sidas have only been tested against cancer 40 times. Every one of them has had significant benefits; many were cytotoxic, apoptotic, etc. Not one study was followed up.
- Sidas protect your liver, kidney & brain (& more), are blood cleansing and help balance your fats/lipids. They are adaptagenic, tonic, aphrodisiac, benefit your digestion, etc.
- There are 160 ways that Sida can benefit you.
- Sida acuta can be grown in Zone 8 outdoors. If you can grow tomatoes, you can probably grow Sida.
- This book is completely based on peer-review research, with some expert testimony.

A User's Guide to Sida acuta, Sida cordifolia, and Sida rhombifolia:: How to Grow, Harvest, and Make the World's Best Herbal Antibiotics, Protein-Rich, Used by Millions, Grow Them Like Tomatoes   48 pp, $6.00 paper, $4.49 Kindle, Book and Sida acuta seeds from the author's site (bbruneau.com) $6.00

This book is for everyone. It tells you how to grow and harvest Sidas, plus the why and how to make essential preparations.